A
CUSHING'S
COLLECTION

A CUSHING'S COLLECTION

A Humorous Journey Surviving Cushing's Disease,
Diabetes Insipidus, and a Bilateral Adrenalectomy

MARIE CONLEY

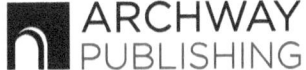

ARCHWAY
PUBLISHING

This book is a work of non-fiction. Unless otherwise noted, the author and the publisher make no explicit guarantees as to the accuracy of the information contained in this book and in some cases, names of people and places have been altered to protect their privacy.

Archway Publishing books may be ordered through booksellers or by contacting:

Archway Publishing
1663 Liberty Drive
Bloomington, IN 47403
www.archwaypublishing.com
1 (888) 242-5904

ISBN: 978-1-4808-2340-2 (sc)
ISBN: 978-1-4808-2341-9 (hc)
ISBN: 978-1-4808-2342-6 (e)

Library of Congress Control Number: 2015917230

Print information available on the last page.

Archway Publishing rev. date: 10/22/2015

Think about getting up, while you are falling down.

~ Joe Paterno

All proceeds from this publication will go to
The Conley Cushing's Disease Fund,
fiscal sponsor The Foundation for Enhancing Communities.
www.kickcushings.com

DEDICATION

This book is dedicated to all Cushing's disease
thrivers. We are a small group but we are mighty.

It is for all of the loved ones of those with Cushing's disease,
because you help make an isolating, rare disease not so lonely.

It is for all of the medical professionals who help
Cushing's disease patients because you have been given
a gift to help make sense out of the nonsensical.

Most especially, it is for my husband, Chris, and
son, Carter, for their love and laughter.

FOREWORD

If you skew the endocrine system, you lose the pathways to self. When endocrine patterns change, it alters the way you think and feel. One shift in the pattern tends to trip another. ~ *Hilary Mantel*

Medical fact: delay to diagnosis in patients with Cushing's disease ranges from 6 months to 10 years. It comes as no surprise that many of my patients have gone through years of medical testing and treatments for many seemingly unrelated illnesses, injuries, and aliments, without finding an elusive unifying cause: Cushing's.

I am fortunate to work at the University of Pennsylvania Hospital Pituitary Center which has a focus on this rare disease. Between two and ten people per million are diagnosed each year with Cushing's which is an endocrine disease.

Because of the disease's individuality and rareness, patients and their families are often left with little information that goes beyond technical aspects of medical testing and treatments.

As a clinician, I am grateful that this publication provides a humorous and insightful look at one of my patient's journey with this disease. Open about her every experience, and determined to overcome it all while helping other Cushing's patients and their families, Marie been an inspiration to all of us: family, friends, other patients and medical professionals alike.

Cushing's disease is just one of many endocrine disorders that are mysterious and isolating but with publications like *A Cushing's Collection*, hopefully my patients and others across the country won't feel so alone.

Julia Kharlip, MD

Associate Medical Director, Penn Pituitary Center
Assistant Professor of Clinical Medicine
Division of Endocrinology, Metabolism and Diabetes

University of Pennsylvania Health System

PREFACE

When I first began e-mailing my friends and family the status reports from my countless doctors' visits, I had no idea the posts would take the shape of a book three years later. However, if I have learned anything since being diagnosed with Cushing's disease, it is how frustrating it was to be deemed an "unusual" case time and time again by each new doctor who stepped into an exam room and picked up my chart. First, my e-mails were intended to educate and inform those closest to me about this disease. Based on the many wonderful responses I received, mission accomplished. If my story – this collection of friendly (and brutally honest) e-mails – can help someone out there recognize various Cushing's symptoms in themselves or others, and shield them from the awful process of being misdiagnosed, then I will have done my job. And if I could be a source of information intertwined with humor and hope for someone's mom, dad, husband, relative or friend who is living with the consequences of Cushing's, then I will feel that this painful journey will have had a true purpose.

Cushing's disease is rare. Some studies between two to ten people per million are affected. Either way, Cushing's IS RARE or it is one of the reasons I went undiagnosed – or misdiagnosed – for so long. Having said that, I will be eternally grateful to my team of doctors and nurses at the Hospital of the University of

Pennsylvania for taking such good care of me once a diagnosis was made. Most especially, I am eternally grateful to my health captain, Dr. Julia Kharlip. She was always kind, compassionate, honest, and there for me during many difficult and scary times. I would be remiss if I did not acknowledge my guardian angel in the form of my certified registered nurse practitioner, Michael Fedor, at Penn State Hershey Medical Group. He has been by my side since day one. He believed in me. He never gave up. He is the constant calm in my life.

As this book began to take shape and I went back and read previous e-mails I had sent to family and friends, I couldn't help but laugh at the absurdity of things I was writing about: hair on my face, a hump on my back, ridiculous acne, fat under my chin. I mean, while these symptoms were happening to me and I didn't know what was causing them, they definitely were NOT funny at the time, but I know I did inject humor into these stories when I first told them because if I didn't, the alternative would have been much worse. So I hope this book guides the reader through an often-unbelievable journey, filled with tears at times, yes, but also with lots of laughter. I will forever be grateful that my sense of humor, a gift from my mom and sister, was alive and well during this mysterious odyssey. This trait blended well with my tenacity, grit, and strength that I got from my dad.

My other objective for turning my collection of e-mails into a book was to leave the reader with hope. At times, I questioned whether it was there, though I mustered it up with God's help when I needed it most. I know He was always there. My wish is for others with Cushing's – those newly diagnosed just beginning their journey – to know that while this can be a scary and frustrating disease due to so many unknowns, it is not a death sentence. They will make it through.

Now that this book is finished, and in your hands, my next goal is to continue raising funds for Cushing's research; so thank you, dear reader, for purchasing this book. All net proceeds of this book will go to The Conley's Cushing's Fund. This fund was established on July 17, 2014 and is a fiscal project of The Foundation for Enhancing Communities. The funds raised will be used in part to create awareness materials for loved ones who are suffering from this disease as well as support institutions and organizations focused on research and treatment of Cushing's disease.

I want to thank the recipients of my many crazy and LONG e-mails about my journey. You never let me thank you for all you did for me, so now I get to do that. I am blessed to be surrounded by such a loving, supportive, and funny group of people.

I want to thank Sue and Scott Paterno for being so patient and compassionate during my illness. Few employers would have been so understanding and I will never forget this. My family and I will never be able to properly articulate what you what you mean to us.

This book would not be possible without the constant love and support of my family, especially my parents, Jean and Chuck, and my sister, Christine, who took care of me in ways I could never have imagined, but am so glad they did.

To my constant, my husband Chris, for helping me off the couch, pushing me up the steps, and loving me no matter what.

Finally to my son, my inspiration, Carter, whose heart and unfiltered honesty and humor, made me feel better on some of the worst days of my life. I love you all so much!

~ *Marie*

INTRODUCTION

I have been called many things in my life but an author was never one of them. So the fact that you are reading something with my name on it is surreal.

My parents raised me to take pride in anything I do and instilled in me the value of a strong work ethic. While at Bloomsburg University, I was involved with our student government and active in my sorority Sigma, Sigma, Sigma. I worked hard and graduated with an appreciation that being part of something bigger than yourself is rare and can shape who you are and who you can be. By coincidence or fate, I volunteered the Tom Ridge for Governor campaign in 1994. It was by working for Governor Tom Ridge, as his scheduler, that I had the privilege of witnessing on a daily basis the importance of being a part of something bigger than you. That one person can make a difference.

Since that time, my career has taken many twists and turns. I worked in Pennsylvania politics for a number of year raising money, helping with stakeholder outreach and messaging. I was a good staffer comfortable behind the scenes. In 2009, I took a huge leap of faith and became the director for a children's' non-profit the Children's Miracle Network at Penn State Hershey Children's Hospital. Working with children at the hospital, our Miracle Children, and their families quickly became one of the most fulfilling and humbling experiences of my life. One quickly gains perspective on what is important in life when you are helping to make a difference in the life of a child when they and their families are hurt and scared. In May 2012, my career took another unique turn and I was asked to start The Paterno Foundation carrying out the priorities of the late Coach Paterno and his wife, Sue focused on education. In December 2012, working with Sue Paterno, her efforts included creating a program for higher education settings on the prevention and awareness of child sexual victimization.

I now realize that God had a reason for my unchartered exciting professional career path for me. I know I am to take all of my experiences, talents, and contacts to help raise awareness for the rare orphan disease I was diagnosed with in June 2012. It is called Cushing's disease and between two and ten people per million are diagnosed a year with it. Through the years, I have worked with such quality individuals that are now in a position to help me create awareness for this disease. My fundraising experience allows me to raise money for The Conley Cushing's Disease Fund, fiscal sponsor The Foundation for Enhancing Communities to support organization and causes that focused on Cushing's disease. This fund will generate opportunities to create awareness materials for family and friends with Cushing's disease as they is so little information available.

This book contains my thoughts and my feelings through my journey. It should not be read as a medical journal. Any endocrine disease is extremely unique to each patient. My stories are simply that <u>my stories</u>. While I know most reading this may share many of the same experiences, medical treatments and test, please remember each person deals with the unknown and healing in different ways. I hope you enjoy my way!

Thank you for sharing this journey with me.

A CUSHING'S COLLECTION:

A Humorous Journey Surviving Cushing's Disease, Diabetes Insipidus, and a Bilateral Adrenalectomy

By Marie Conley

From: Marie Conley
Sent: Monday, June 04, 2012 5:33 PM
Subject: Moon Face, Buffalo Hump, and test OH MY!

Hey, all! First, thank you so much for calling and e-mailing about my appointment on Friday. I am sorry I have not been more responsive and am just getting back to all of you now, but I think you will be interested to read this latest post.

I spent two hours with the endocrinologist (fourth specialist since February) from the University of Pennsylvania on Friday afternoon. She was very kind and thorough; she reviewed all of my paperwork and did an examination. She was not able to say conclusively what the heck this is. However, what I am being tested for *this* week is called Cushing's disease. I will have a series of tests that will determine if this is what I have; results will likely take three to four weeks.

I am not going to focus on what could or could not be until I get the results. I will share, however, that this is the first thing that makes sense. Of the eleven most prominent symptoms, I have at least nine of them. While I have not been nuts researching, everything is pointing to Cushing's.

Just as an aside, of course, I will probably have the disease with the symptoms called "Moon Face" and "Buffalo Hump!" For the record, "Moon Face" is a swollen face - prominently bloated under the chin in the neck region (for those of you who haven't seen me lately I look like the Stay Puft Marshmallow Man from *Ghostbusters*) and "Buffalo Hump" is a collection of fat on the back at the base of the neck. Ladies, watch your men - I am very sexy right now!

Other goodies include: increased weight gain (nineteen pounds since March 1 even though I have worked out six days a week - ran a 10K race and a sprint Triathlon and ate #(*@&#(@ red peppers and carrots for dessert), red face, acne, abdominal swelling, and bone thinning (had the stress fracture and now have another tear in my hip).

The most important thing is, if this is Cushing's disease, it is not hereditary and Carter is fine and will never get what I have! While I am still uncomfortable, I am not in pain and can take care of Carter, Chris, our home, and my work. I am very lucky that I have my dad's tenacity and I will fight hard until I have all the answers!

I am just so grateful that there may finally be a light at the end of this twelve month tunnel.

I cannot thank you enough for your friendship and thoughts. Please understand if I am not the most visible person in the next couple of months; I am honestly not very comfortable being in public. I don't look like myself.

I have not shared this with a lot of people so I would appreciate that, until I know something, you not share this with anyone (unless you overhear someone say "OHMYGOD, did you see how big Marie Conley got?" Then I am totally comfortable with you printing out this e-mail and sharing it!!! - Just kidding (not really)! I promise to keep you posted when I hear something.

Love, Me!

From: Marie Conley
Sent: Friday, July 13, 2012 11:22 PM
Subject: Update

I apologize that this is all in a long e-mail, and for some, may be the first time I am reaching out about this. As most of you know, I have had a funky, unexplained swelling starting in my legs since last May. It became progressively worse throughout the year moving to my arms and face. Since December 2011, I have seen several specialists and doctors (ten to be exact) and thought there was a course of action. In late April, I sought, another opinion at the University of Pennsylvania. This specialist did not feel that he could treat me, was concerned about my symptoms, and referred me to another specialist, an endocrinologist, Dr. Julia Kharlip.

In early June, Dr. Kharlip and I met and reviewed my symptoms. After weeks of testing, I was FINALLY diagnosed with something called Cushing's disease. This is a very rare condition that affects fewer than 3,000 people a year. I have a benign tumor on my pituitary gland, which is located in the middle of the brain.

It causes my body to secrete an insane amount of cortisol (steroids) throughout my body.

To give you a quick Cushing's 101, the pituitary gland (the master gland) is responsible for:

Regulating blood sugar, maintaining metabolism, controlling reproductive messaging between the brain and organs, and, breaking down fats, proteins, and carbohydrates. The pituitary also supports your immune system and works with your kidneys to maintain proper sodium levels and break down your sugars. In effect, the gland functions as a thermostat that controls all other glands that are responsible for hormone secretion.

While we will never be certain, the doctors think I have probably had this since May 2010. It explains the following things that have occurred to me since then: four rounds of bronchitis, pneumonia, strep, shingles, a fractured hip, a current new hip injury (bone brittleness is a common symptom of Cushing's – I am not allowed to do anything for fear of a bone fracture), and an umbilical hernia and foot problem that both need surgery.

It also explains all of the sexy symptoms I have which are attributed to Cushing's disease: "Moon Face," "Buffalo Hump," (seriously, that is the medical term for it!) unexplained weight gain/obesity of the torso, (even though I trained for and finished a 10K race, half marathon, two sprint-triathlons, and several 5K's during this time frame) a red face, and facial hair. (Having conferred with my agent, I will not be on the runway this fall during Fashion Week).

While my doctor said this is probably not a consolation now, I am lucky to have been so persistent as this disease is very difficult to diagnose and usually takes years to do so. I am not in pain. And while I am very uncomfortable, I can function as a mother, wife, and an employee.

My course of treatment begins on Friday, August third. I will have brain surgery at the Hospital of the University of Pennsylvania to remove the tumor. The procedure will take about four hours and the surgeons will be able to perform the surgery through my nose so I will not be losing my hair!!!! Six surgical teams in the country perform this procedure. I am SO lucky that one is at HUP. I then begin a treatment plan that will continue over the next six to twelve months. It will take time to "teach" my pituitary gland to act *normally* again. Unbelievably, the doctors have shared that the easy part of this is the actual surgery. I have full faith and trust in my doctors.

I will be in the hospital for about four days and will stay close to the hospital for another three to five days before heading back home. Once I am back in Hershey, I will be homebound for about a month to avoid infection. I am very lucky that I now work from home so I will be able to perform as normally. I have only been working for Sue Paterno and her family for four weeks before my diagnosis, they have been nothing but supportive and work is helping me heal (and cope)!

If you are receiving this e-mail, it is because I want you to hear this from **me**. This disease is so rare and there is very little legitimate information out there about it. As a family, we understand how serious this is but we caught it early (relatively speaking) and have a plan of action and attack.

The hardest part will be telling Carter. But I think once we share that HUP has a better ice cream selection in their cafeteria then Penn State Hershey has, all will be right with the world! We plan to tell him as we get closer to the surgery date.

We will get through this as we only know how… with humor and God's help. Chris is already blaming Cushing's for all the times he swears "he told me something" as Cushing's can cause forgetfulness. (He will be milking that one for a while.) He also has a million jokes about the facial hair.

I am sorry for the length of this e-mail but I wanted to make sure you knew what was going on. You know how facts get all crazy and distorted. Lord knows by the time you read this, I could be getting a lobotomy by a mad scientist in New Guinea.

We cannot thank you enough for all your well wishes and kind thoughts. I will make sure Chris e-mails you after the surgery to let you know everything is AOK!

Lastly, while I do not expect you to watch this, below is a great four-minute piece on Cushing's disease produced by *National Geographic*. Who knows, maybe the next time you play Trivial Pursuit, Cushing's might be an answer to a final question!

http://www.youtube.com/watch?v=vxSAhLyKVqw

Author's note: This is a link to a National Geographic piece on Cushing's syndrome.

From: Marie Conley
Sent: Thursday, August 02, 2012 4:41 PM
Subject: Cushing's Alert

To my ladies:

I wanted to take a moment to thank each of you for your support over these past seven weeks. It certainly has been interesting. Your phone calls, cards, texts, and e-mails have meant more to me than you know. (I am sorry if I haven't returned calls this week.) Regardless of how you entered my life, you are truly in my heart. I am blessed.

You have laughed appropriately at my inappropriate jokes, held my hand when tears came to my eyes, made me laugh when I needed it, and encouraged me to let people in and help.

We go in tomorrow at **5:30 am** (please let the surgical staff have their caffeine by then). We are staying at Penn Tower tonight; that is the hotel connected to the Hospital.

Chris will e-mail everything after the surgery. Don't be surprised if I am e-mailing later, too.

I have received some amazing inspirational words of encouragement. Between "Moon Face" and my lovely hump, I needed it! I wanted to share with you the song I will have with me as I move into surgery!

Please click on the link and go to 1:32 seconds - it is just a few seconds long!

http://www.youtube.com/watch?v=cj9_yW8tZxs

Author's note: This is a link to 1990's Hip Hop Group, Digital Underground and their hit song: Humpty Hump Dance.

Send good vibes and prayers!

PS: We told Carter on Sunday. He wanted to take the picture of the MRI to camp so he could show everyone my brains. He said the doctor should go in through my ear - it is closer to my brain than the nose. He will be putting me through "challenges" (thank you Wii) when I get home to test my energy levels - 0 through 10. Finally, he wanted to know if the hospital had Choco Taco ice cream?

From: Marie Conley
Sent: Friday, August 03, 2012 1:17 PM
Subject: Update

First, thank you so much already for your prayers, well wishes, and good vibes.

Marie went into surgery this morning at 5:30 am. She was under for six hours and the surgeons are pleased with how everything went.

We will know if the surgery was successful within the next 48 hours.

She will be in the IUC for at least the next 24 hours and then should be moved into a room. The doctors say the next 24 - 48 hours could be a little crappy as her body realizes it doesn't have any cortisol (steroids) being produced. As the doctors have explained it, her body was drowning in cortisol so it will be an adjustment.

Assuming no complications, she will be at the University of Pennsylvania until Monday.

She will then be at her parents until Sunday. Her parents live about 40 minutes from the Hospital and the doctors want her close to them and an ER for five to seven days post-surgery. Assuming everything is fine, she will be back at home Monday, August 13.

We are going to try to have Carter visit tomorrow or Sunday depending on how things go. He has taken this amazingly well. He wanted to take the picture of the MRI to camp to show everyone his mom's brains. He asked if there were Choco Taco (ice cream treat) at this hospital, so clearly our priorities are in order!

It will come as no surprise to any of you if you start getting e-mails or texts from Marie within the next couple of days.

Thank you again for everything and we will keep you posted if there are any major changes.

From: Marie Conley
Sent: Monday, August 06, 2012 4:44 PM
Subject: Marie Update 2

Hi! Greetings from University of Pennsylvania ICU! I am still here and will be in the hospital until Wednesday. Clearly, someone did not read the memo that I was to be at my parents today resting and no longer in the hospital.

Chris and I wanted to thank you all so much for your prayers and outreach. As you read from Chris's e-mail on Friday, the surgery went well. I have been experiencing a few complications with my kidneys, which is not completely unusual. The doctors are having some difficulty remedying it because my symptoms continue to change - hence the extended stay in the ICU. The neurosurgeon had to manipulate my pituitary gland quite a bit during surgery and it clearly made the gland angry, and it is now reacting. The great news is my cortisol levels are going down and that is a great sign that the surgery was a success.

They continue to do labs and cultures and will get this cleared up soon. In the interim, I am hanging in there. I will be candid and say it is a little rougher than I thought, but in the grand picture, this is nothing! I am just excited to have some energy right now!

The goal is to have me out of the ICU by tomorrow afternoon, in the "step-down" ward tomorrow night, and at my parents on Wednesday.

I will keep you posted! Thank you again for everything!

From: Marie Conley
Sent: Wednesday, August 08, 2012 1:59 PM
Subject: Marie Update 2

Hey all. You guys are the best - your e-mails and texts mean a lot and I feel your prayers. Chris and I are very lucky.

I am still in the ICU and they are having some difficulty figuring out what to do next about my kidney outputs! It is very frustrating because I feel good but these kidney things are pretty important.

We received some disappointing news Monday evening and it was confirmed yesterday. The surgery has not worked the way it was supposed to. I will share that it has been a difficult 24 hours. While the cortisol levels have dropped significantly, they are not in the "cured" range; therefore, the surgery was unsuccessful. In fact, the cortisol levels continue to fluctuate. It was a lot to comprehend and while no decisions can be made for another five weeks, both the neurosurgeon and my endocrinologist agree that we are going to need to look at other options. The surgery has an 85 percent success rate. Guess who's in the fifteen percentile? (Surprise, surprise)

There are a couple of options possible, but more than likely, I will need to have my adrenal glands removed. These are glands that sit atop my kidneys. (Don't worry; I will educate you if this is what is going to happen). If they do have to remove them, my hope is they are 10 pounds each and I will be on my way to losing this weight.

SO, I head back on the Turnpike to Hershey in a few days (hopefully) after a five-hour brain surgery, six days in the ICU, blood draws every three hours, injections in my stomach, seven IV lines, heart monitors, kidney issues, the worst stuffed up nose EVER, and the ugliest hospital gown with my butt shown to the world. Plus, I can't drive, can't lift anything over ten pounds, AND I still will have all of the symptoms I had when I left. (OK that is my only pity party).

I'll keep you posted. I will send an e-mail to the larger group next week once I am settled. I am sure you can understand that it is still kind of raw, so feel free, if anyone asks, to share. It is one less person I have to tell the story to. Peace out...

From: Marie Conley
Sent: Thursday, August 16, 2012 11:15 PM
Subject: Marie Update

It is not often that you get to find out just how lucky you are to have such great friends and family. Over the past two weeks, the outpouring of well wishes and support has humbled Chris and me as we have managed through this craziness. Carter has been an absolute champ during this whole process - we are in awe of him.

I finally arrived back home to Hershey yesterday after nine long days in the ICU at HUP. Technically, the brain surgery went well, though we could not get my kidneys and pituitary gland to work together until late Sunday night.

Unfortunately, we received some difficult news last week. The surgery was not successful. My Cushing's disease and all of its glorious symptoms are still ever present. I have no regrets as this procedure has an eighty-five percent success rate. I am in that ugly fifteen percent. My doctors and nurses were amazing, and having seen some of the patients that were on my floor, I realize I am still a very lucky person. There is a rare exception called a "delayed" response that could happen in a six-week window post-surgery, but neither my neurosurgeon nor my endocrinologist is particularly hopeful.

Chris and I will meet my doctor again Sept. 11 to figure out our next steps. This unique disease affects fewer than 3,000 people a year. There are not many additional options for treatment: another try at the brain surgery, radiation therapy, or removal of the adrenal glands (they are located atop the kidneys). We need to continue to move forward because, as was the case before the surgery, the cortisol continues to wreak havoc to almost every area of my body.

For the next three weeks, I am homebound recovering from the surgery. As you can imagine, my patience and temperament clearly will support no driving. I can lift no more than five pounds, and to reduce the chance of infection, I cannot go out in public.

We appreciate you keeping us in your thoughts and we will keep you posted once we have decided what is the best course of action to get me healthy.

This time next year, I will be a few weeks away from running in the Hershey Half Marathon!

From: Marie Conley
Sent: Monday, September 17, 2012 9:45 AM
Subject: Marie Update

We cannot thank you enough for all of the outreach since I came home from the hospital. This is another long e-mail but I want to make sure you have a full and complete understanding of what is going on. I truly apologize if I have not returned calls or e-mails; I am just trying to get my arms around all of this. My way of dealing with this right now is being with Chris and Carter and powering through with work.

Chris and I went to see many doctors this past week at the University of Pennsylvania Hospital to try to figure out our next steps.

Recognizing the rarity of this disease, being informed that my cortisol (steroid) and other levels are higher now than they were when I was diagnosed in June, and knowing the limited options of treating this disease, we knew this was going to be a difficult couple of days.

There are four options for treatment after a failed brain surgery for Cushing's disease patients:

1) Try the brain surgery again – after speaking with my neurosurgeon, this is not a good option for me. There is no visible tumor so they would have to remove my entire pituitary gland and the risk of the symptoms returning is 50 percent. I would be on four medicines for the rest of my life. (I would also be kicked into early menopause; Chris nixed this option right away)

2) Radiation – this is not an option for me as it generally takes two to five years for the symptoms to alleviate.

3) Medicinal therapy – There are no real medicines that exist that can completely address Cushing's disease long-term with significant results.

4) Adrenalectomy – Complete removal of your adrenal glands. While this is a very serious step, it is not unusual for this disease. This surgery stops the symptoms immediately and while I will always have the disease, the

symptoms of Cushing's disease could no longer return. I would be on two medicines for the rest of my life.

I have decided to undergo an adrenalectomy Oct. 8 at the University of Pennsylvania. Chris and I have full confidence in my doctors and surgeons, and the pros outweigh the cons. (Carter does not know anything yet. We are going to let him know the week before, just like last time.)

Quick biology lesson (from the person who hated biology): You have two adrenal glands that sit atop of your kidneys. They are responsible for producing really important things like adrenaline and other hormones necessary to keep a fluid and electrolyte (salt) balance in the body. They are also responsible for producing and pushing out the appropriate cortisol levels to address all of the functions controlled by the pituitary gland. (i.e. immune system, bone brittleness, metabolism, and so much more)

As I understand it, I will always have Cushing's disease but this may be the only way to stop the symptoms. The cells left over in my brain that have been sending the messages to the adrenal glands after the surgery to release the crazy amount of cortisol will always be there. However, by removing the adrenal glands, we are removing the receivers of the message. I will always have to monitor the "cells" in my brain but this is relatively easy and painless.

It is a little funny because I think they are taking this surgery a little more seriously than the brain surgery. Unfortunately, with Cushing's disease, your immune system is severely suppressed, risk of infection is higher, and you can bleed more easily in surgery. The doctors shared that it is hard to determine the damage this disease has done to my organs and glands until they are in there. No offense –brain surgery still sounds a lot scarier.

The adrenalectomy will be done laparoscopically and will take about five hours. The best part is my surgeon will fix my umbilical hernia on the "way out." (Now if I could only find a way to sneak my podiatrist into the room to fix my foot…) They say I should be in the hospital three days, then home (heard that before…) I will be unable to drive for about a week or two. All physical activity will be curbed big time for about eight weeks. I was hoping each adrenal gland was about 20 pounds each so I would be on my way to losing this weight; unfortunately, they are only a couple ounces each!

We are back where we started in my original e-mail in July. The doctors say the weird thing about this disease is that the easy part is the surgery; the challenging part is the months following. It can take the body a long time to adjust to no longer having any cortisol. Because of removing the adrenal glands, I will have to get used to not having a natural adrenaline surge. The great news is my medicines will assist with both of these functions. Good way to think of it is - I wake up every morning with a tank of gas, I will draw down from that tank throughout the day – when I am done – I am done! I need to work with my doctors on how to make sure (with the medicine) my tank stays full throughout the day. There is no reason not to believe that the quality of life I want and yearn for again will return after all of this stuff is figured out.

After weighing all of this, my two greatest concerns were the following:

- First, the complication I had after the first surgery with my kidneys is permanent. I have to take a medicine nightly to help with this. I thought I would be unable to drink alcohol while on the medicine. This was unacceptable and a possible deal breaker. I have "Moon Face,"

"Buffalo Hump" (although now it seems like an elephant hump) and insane weight gain AND now you want to take away alcohol – Hell NO! I have verified that, in fact, I CAN drink socially with this medicine.

- Second, I am not, nor have I ever, been a jewelry person. I now have to wear one of those medical bracelets every day for the rest of my life. I refuse to wear one of those ugly things! Thank God, someone else feels the same way and there are websites of "designer" medical bracelets and watches for me to purchase.

Clearly, my priorities are set!

We appreciate your prayers – we need them! We have learned every time a doctor says, "This is rare, unique or we don't often see this" – it seems to happen to me. We need God's help to get this right.

Chris will send an e-mail out after the surgery to let you know all is AOK! Thank you again for all of your support, help, humor, and compassion through this all. This time next year, this will have been a blip in my life and I will be two weeks out from running the Hershey Half Marathon...can't wait!

From: Marie Conley
Sent: Saturday, September 29, 2012 8:12 PM
Subject: Dear Diary…

Dear Diary,

It has been a crazy couple of weeks. Chris and I came to a decision three weeks ago on how to best deal with this disease and the surgery is one week away. My friends and family have been amazing but I think most are ready to kill me because I have pretty much been MIA.

Last week, I spoke to a woman, Fabiana, who has Cushing's disease and is a patient of my doctors. Her first brain surgery was about ten years ago. Her symptoms came back last year and she had the brain surgery again in October of 2011. It failed. She had the adrenalectomy in January. I am forever grateful that we spoke. It was the first time I was able to have someone finish my sentences and understand everything I have experienced. She made what is about to happen to me VERY real. I knew what was ahead of me was not going to be easy and she confirmed this. I am also more prepared for the pain and sickness that will happen after the surgery and the weeks following. I asked my mom to stay with me for the week (s) after the surgery per Fabiana's advice. My doctor prepared me for this prior to the brain surgery but it quickly passed when the surgery failed. It also means something completely different when you are speaking with someone who has gone through it. She and I plan to stay in touch.

I also decided to go to the Pennsylvania State Chamber dinner on Monday night. I was excited to go because James Carville and Karl Rove were the speakers. I ended up coming home so depressed for a couple of reasons. The problems with my kidneys made me have to get up and go to the bathroom so many times. Worse, no one really talked to me the way they used to... it was all about being sick. Even worse, some people didn't even know who I was! I was on this guy's campaign for six months, I went to his daughter's basketball game with him and his wife, but he didn't recognize me. Then I had to tell him what happened because he didn't know what to say. This happened more times than I could count!

So with the conversation with Fabiana, the dinner, an increased pants size in just three weeks, the realization that I will not be able to do much for at least eight weeks post-surgery, the stress on my family, shortness of breath, the impact on my professional career, and not being able to walk well and always in pain – I cracked. This past week I finally broke. I had a good cry. I think it was healthy! I think it all finally caught up to me. It is outta' me now and I am refocused and ready to kick butt!

Diary, I hope my friends realize how much they mean to me and how I know, I could not do this alone. I think they also know I would probably **never** share any of the stuff that I wrote with them because I am me and if I did I would probably end up crying. I hope they know I am not trying to be rude or unresponsive - I am just trying to cope.

So I am so glad I have my diary to write in... wouldn't it be funny if somehow this diary entry ended up in an e-mail...

Love you all!

PS: We head down the shore on Friday then will travel up to Philadelphia on Sunday night to stay with my sister. Christy is going to take Carter around the city on Monday during my surgery. I won't find out what time my surgery is until Friday night - I will e-mail you the time when I get it. It will more than likely be early because it is a five to six hour surgery.

From: Marie Conley
Sent: Monday, October 8, 2012 5:37 PM
Subject: Marie Update

Thank you for your words of support leading up to today. We arrived at the hospital around 5:30 am and just like Gilligan's Island it was much more than a 3 hour tour. Marie's surgery went very well and there were no complications with the removal of her two adrenal glands. However, she did experience large fluctuations of both her blood pressure and heart rate. After roughly 4 hours of surgery, they decided to end the surgery with only removing her adrenal glands and as a result addressing the umbilical hernia will have to occur in the future after Marie's body heals from the surgery and stabilizes with the steroid replacement regimen.

The next couple days will be a little difficult as her body adjusts to the new levels of cortisol and lack of naturally produced adrenaline. It is as if her body will be going through withdraw, similar to what someone who is addicted to drugs would experience. Over the next few days, the doctors will work to stabilize Marie's steroid levels through drugs as though her body was naturally producing the steroids at "healthy" levels. Assuming things progress as planned, she will be home in Hershey by the end of the week. The next couple weeks will be a little challenging for Marie as she adjusts to her "new normal." She will be dealing with a lot of fatigue and adjustments with medications. She will not be able to drive for about two weeks and can't do any strenuous activity for about eight weeks.

Carter spent the day exploring Philadelphia with his Aunt Christy (the Franklin Institute and the Dinosaur exhibit and the Academy of Natural Sciences) and is returning home tonight with his Pop-Pop to prepare for school the rest of the week. He has handled this like a trooper and is so strong.

Marie will reach out to everyone later in the week.

Hopefully this begins the road (albeit long) to recovery. Thank you again for all of your love, friendship, and support!

Chris

From: Lauren Cotter Brobson
Sent: Wednesday, October 10, 2012 2:17 PM
Subject: Marie Update

Ladies:

I spoke with Marie briefly this morning. She asked that I write all of you — her closest circle of support. First, she wants to say thank you for all of your kind words and messages. I think you all received the general update that went out post-surgery. She asked that I share with you, a much smaller group, and the developments over the last two days.

The headline is that she is experiencing what was to be expected -- post-op pain and a body that is trying once again to reboot itself, this time without the adrenal glands. In typical Marie Conley fashion, there is not a straight path from here to there.

You might remember that one of the side effects of the brain surgery was her kidneys kicking into overtime and putting her urine output into high gear. Well, yesterday, her body didn't produce enough urine. Instead, her sodium levels skyrocketed and her body retained too much water. She was very swollen and as a result, very sore and limited in her movements (like the ability to even grasp a utensil). They had to put her on some oxygen to help ease her breathing; again, because of the pressure her body is putting on itself. This is a temporary situation, but obviously very uncomfortable. Her endocrinologist is "on it" and whatever meds they gave her late last night seemed to be working some-what as she had some relief this morning. Hopefully today will see more progress with that. She really just needs to keep rest-ing and keep up with her pain management (they gave her the self-directed drip (YEAH!) so her body can do its job and heal.

Marie amazingly remains determined and forward thinking. I don't know how she does it... but that is why and how we all love her.

Once again, some super-sensitive fellowship student, who missed the day the professor talked about bedside manners, made some remark about what an unusual case she is... Lovely. But I do find comfort in knowing that she is at U Penn and get-ting the best possible care there.

I will keep you updated, as I receive additional info. I am back in Harrisburg right now making sure Carter has some sense of normal. Marie's parents and sister are providing bedside enter-tainment and company. When she needs us, she will let us know what she needs us to do...right now, her request is to send all of our prayers and good thoughts her way.

Author note: E-mail was printed with the permission of Lauren Cotter Brosbon, a close family friend.

From: Marie Conley
Sent: Thursday, October 11, 2012 7:51 PM
Subject: Joe, Paul, and an open-backed gown

... What more could a gal ask for? There was a silly rumor among the hospital staff that I would be bustin' outta' here today but I knew better. When one of my surgeons came in to discuss my discharge, she didn't like what she saw on two of the eight inci-sions on my belly. She literally circled them with her pen (My mom was there; she saw it.) Literally the pen she wrote out my prescriptions with – BOOM- wrote right on my skin and ordered two doses of IV antibiotics for this afternoon and tomorrow morning, and just like that, I am still here. I told anyone who would listen that until I was in my parents' car on I-95 headed north, I would not get excited about leaving.

The swelling has gone down a little and my medicines seem to be regulating themselves. I was told I probably urinated about nine pounds yesterday. (Note: there is no excitement on my part, as it doesn't make a lick of difference other than I found my ankles again and I do in fact have five fingers and not sausages at the end of my hands now).

My mother and sister have proven to be caring, loving, and patient caregivers and have taken care of me in ways that they should not have to. Chris has been amazing at keeping Carter happy and not worried and keeping me focused on the end goal. And my dad is making sure there is enough food to nourish me when I get back to their home tomorrow and keeping us all on task. My friend Elizabeth, who is the librarian at Carter's school, said everyone is keeping an eye on him and making sure he is okay. And of course, all of you, sending funny texts and e-mails and leaving voice mail messages - this has gotten me through thus far.

As you can expect, there are a couple of great stories to come from this but I think they are better told by Chris and my mom. Needless to say, I apologized to everyone I came in contact with on Monday between 2:30 pm - 6 pm as I do not recall one conversation. Ya' know how friends don't let friends drink and drive? Moms, sisters and husbands should not let friends DUIA (Dial Under the Influence of Anesthesia). I apparently called my endocrinologist's office and told the receptionist that "I am in my room and there is no medicine regimen and the nurses don't know what they are supposed to do and how was she going to fix it!"

I hope to be discharged by noon tomorrow and back to my parents' home tomorrow afternoon. My mom and I head back to Hershey on Saturday morning.

So, it is another glorious night at HUP but I am breathing, laughing, and on the way to recovery. And I swear I can see my cheekbones for real and my face is almost flesh colored and not red -- how cool.

So tonight, I am joined with Joe Biden and Paul Ryan and will try to solve the world's problems from room 1228.

Can't wait to see you all.

PS: I finally got smart and asked for a sleeping pill tonight.

From: Marie Conley
Sent: Sunday, October 14, 2012 10:11 PM
Subject: Marie's Last Update

I am so happy to say this should be my last e-mail correspondence to you about my health. I was discharged from the hospital on Friday and returned home on Saturday. While it is only 96 miles on the turnpike from Philly to Hershey, the journey to get here seemed much longer.

On behalf of Chris, Carter, and myself, thank you so much for all you have done to make this journey a little easier. Your support, humor, friendship, culinary treats, calls, gifts, e-mails, and most especially prayers allowed our family to survive this odd time.

As Chris shared earlier in the week, the operation was success-ful. I experienced a few complications (big surprise) while in the hospital but thanks to my amazing doctors and nurses, all is well.

It is hard to believe that on July 13, I shared that I was diagnosed with a crazy rare disease called Cushing's. Through my e-mails, you came to understand the unusual course of treatment, the challenges we experienced as a family with a failed brain sur-gery, and the decisions we needed to make to get this sickness under control.

Four months and one day from the day of my diagnosis, I am now minus one brain tumor, two adrenal glands and I have added a host of daily medications that will help to keep me healthy for the rest of my life. I will admit I would have the brain surgery again in a heartbeat over the bilateral adrenalectomy. I finally found the one thing that can slow me down... eight incisions in my stomach. I am pretty much homebound (and helpless) for the next two weeks. My body is adjusting to these new medications and healing from both surgeries. My mother, my guardian angel, is staying with us.

This disease has taught me so much. The two most valuable things are how important it is to appreciate all that I have been given and how blessed I am to have such a great circle of family and friends. One of the most challenging aspects of this disease, even after having two major surgeries, is what lies ahead in the next few weeks to 12 months. We know we could not do this without our circle of support.

Because of the love and compassion of my friends and family, the Paterno family's support of me both professionally and per-sonally, and the dedicated and tenacious team of doctors and nurses at University of Pennsylvania hospital, I know I have the fortitude needed to continue to fight.

So it is with a great deal of happiness that I am signing off and trying to begin what will now be my "new normal." I know the journey ahead is not easy but each bump in the road will make me stronger. Thank you again for making this voyage doable. You have helped me turn fears, frustration, and tears into courage, conviction, and laughter.

I hope no one you know ever has to go through this, but I do feel that through this experience, there is now a population of people who are educated about this disease. Maybe someday, you will be able to help someone because you traveled this road with me. Remember, fewer than 10 in one million people a year are diagnosed with Cushing's disease and it usually takes three to ten years for an accurate diagnosis. You could help change those numbers!

So here is to a healthier tomorrow!

From: Marie Conley
Sent: Monday, October 15, 2012 1:04 PM
Subject: My ladies

I have you now in my own separate category called my "cushette's." As you saw from my earlier e-mail, I am trying to close the loop on the larger group. I hope that people will just start to think of me again as the assertive, stubborn Marie Conley and not the sick Marie Conley. However, as my closest peeps, I will continue to update you all on what is going on. As I have shared, the next months ahead will be the crappiest and that frightens me more than any of the surgeries did.

My only focus this week is on getting better so I can make Carter's Race for Education Relay on Friday morning. I also have to just bite the bullet and order the stupid, ugly medical alert bracelet. I feel like crap and am not sure if is the aftermath of the surgery, medications, anxiety, or a mixture of everything. I am told I will probably feel like this for at least three weeks. I have follow-up appointments next Wednesday in Philly.

I will continue to rely on all of you for my strength when I need it and I know I can ask for it. I will also share triumphs, frustrations, and ironies. Speaking of ironies...

The only symptom of Cushing's I have embraced was the absence of my period since December. On Friday late morning, I am discharged. Trooper Chuck (my dad) is carefully driving up I-95N trying to avoid potholes and bumps (HA HA). We get in the house after hitting CVS and picking up more medicines than my 87-year- old grandmother uses. I cautiously go to the bathroom and BAM - my freaking period. Really?

I couldn't get rid of a little "Moon Face" or even the acne – nope, but the period is back in full force! (Ha Ha, God, very funny)

I would love to have some visitors next week if anyone wants to travel!

Love you all!

From: Marie Conley
Sent: October 26, 2012
Subject: My ladies

Hey ladies:

I hope you are all well. I am heading into week three post-op and feeling better each day. I can get around much better – slower, but better. I can see a little difference each day. My face isn't as red and Chris has noticed that my posture has improved. I am not out of breath walking up the steps and my hips don't hurt either; I am excited.

My mom stayed with me until this past Tuesday and she came with me to my appointment with my endocrinologist. I had several questions prepared for Dr. Kharlip regarding the next few months. She explained everything so well and was realistic as to what I should expect as my body adjusts to all of this! What was interesting was that each cell in your body needs some amount of cortisol. Over the next few months, my cells will learn to adjust to the new "normal" levels. Once this happens, my cells will start acting normally and I will start to break down proteins, sugars, and carbohydrates the normal way. My bone "cells" will start to become stronger again. The damaged internal tissue will start to heal, etc. It is really kind of cool.

- Over the course of the next three months, I will need to adjust my medications every two weeks to start to lower my hydrocortisone (aka my fake cortisol). The doctor was very honest that we, as a family, will need to prepare for each adjustment. I will need to be prepared to feel pretty yucky and be in bed for two days following each new dose of medicine. It will be like the flu with aches and pains and I will be crazy tired.

- Dr. Kharlip is very concerned about the bone brittleness component. I need to work with a physical therapist to start to assess my strength (or rather lack of strength.) With most Cushing's disease patients, you start with core strengthening but because of my hernia that will be a little tricky. I will also need an assessment to see if my upper body can sustain crutches so I can get my foot fixed. My podiatrist said that I would need to be on crutches for at least two weeks. I personally think I am in pretty good shape. Because I trained for the 10K and Tri in May, I am a lot stronger than most Cushing's disease patients are. Up until the brain surgery, I was able to walk about 45 minutes a day so I am hoping I am not too bad off!

— I am starting to play with my medicine that helps regulate "output." I haven't properly explained this lovely permanent condition, called Diabetes insipidus (DI). It is a result of the brain surgery and creates excessive thirst and excretion of large amounts of severely diluted urine (told ya' it was lovely); It can actually be somewhat serious because your body has to have a balanced amount of electrolytes and sodium to function properly; It will hopefully start allowing me to be a normal person again from the timeframe of 5:30pm – 10:00 pm (i.e. not drinking every liquid in sight and not going to the bathroom four times an hour)

— I asked the doctor about the cognitive challenges that I sometimes experience and she said that not only did I have major brain surgery less than ten weeks ago but I was under anesthesia for over eleven hours in fewer than two and half months. She said that those drugs are crazy strong and have an impact on the brain. I told her I was on two conference calls on Monday and she was not happy. Needless to say, she would like to see me resting (I told her that I was really proud of myself because, for me, I really am resting). She told me to be patient.

The good news is my surgeon, Dr. Fraker, has agreed to do my hernia surgery. He normally would never do anything this "simple" but because of my Cushing's and the tendency for weird things to happen to me, he will do it; it will be sometime in March.

So it was a TON to digest – I think my mom was a little taken aback (Mom, feel free to comment or e-mail anything I have missed). I got a little sad and felt a little sorry for myself for a couple hours about what the next six months will be like, but then I just decided to say "eff it" and continue to beat this thing.

Chris and Carter have been great. Carter continues to monitor how much I can lift and yells at me when it is more than five pounds. He thinks my eight incisions are really cool and would like me to lift my shirt to show people! Chris continues to be my rock. We could not have made it through the past two weeks without my parents, especially my mom.

So, that is it for now. I cannot wait to see you all and catch up in person!

Love, me!

From: Marie Conley
Sent: Monday, November 19, 2012 9:50 AM
Subject: Marie update

So, I was thinking at 3:00 am on Saturday morning, how can I get myself into one of those sexy scratchy butt-baring hospital gowns? What can I do to have that feeling again of a one-inch gage needle in my vein only to have it pop and replaced again?? Wait, I know...I will make myself start vomiting and won't stop for thirteen hours so I can go back into the ER and be admitted for two days!

Yes, my friends, my master plan worked. I am writing to you from Room 6262 at Penn State Hershey Medical Center wearing a stylish cotton, starred dress with my butt hanging out and steroids coursing through my veins!

I came in Saturday around 2:00 pm and they admitted me by 6:00 pm. I pretty much knew, even though they wouldn't say it, that I was going to be stuck here on Sunday night, too. (Secretly I wanted to because tonight's dinner is baked ham with pineapple "toppings"- what else can a girl ask for?). I had severe nausea and vomiting, a killer headache, and body aches and cramps - classic signs of adrenal failure and/or problems with the cortisol/steroid levels. My sodium level was 122. It is supposed to be around 139-145. My doctor likes it at 140.

The nurse kept coming in wanting to make sure I was ok, not disoriented etc.

Finally she explained that when numbers get that low it is often accompanied with severe disorientation, aggression, confusion. (I will pause now for all of your jokes.....) She actually couldn't believe I was talking and still writing down notes in my trusty four-inch Cushing's Binder.

"Faster than a speeding bullet, more powerful than a locomotive, able to do Sprint-Tri's in a single bound (because I have insane amounts of steroids coursing through my veins) and survive low sodium levels..." It's a "Moon Face." It's a "Buffalo Hump." No, it's Super-Cushing's!

The awesome doctors at Penn State Hershey have been working with my doctors at University of Pennsylvania and they are working on a plan. As expected, it is not easy to figure out what caused this but there are a host of medical reasons that are boring and complicated. Chances are my numbers will be in the normal range by tonight and they will need to make sure they stabilize for twelve hours, then, I am outta' here. My docs kept emphasizing prior to the surgeries that they, the surgeries, are the easy part of treating this disease. It is the months following that are difficult. So suffice it to say, it is all good!

I will say Carter took this one a little harder. We think it is starting to get to him, how could it not? He started crying that he wanted to come to the hospital with us because he was old enough to understand. We allowed him to stay an hour to let him be a part of this. He got scared and started to cry a little in the hospital and quickly said " I don't know why I am crying ; it must be my allergies." I assured him that my allergies were really bad in here, too, and that's why my eyes were teary!

His Nana and Pops Ted picked him up and then they did the heroic task of taking him to the annual school Spaghetti Dinner. Then Chris made things all good in the world for him again so life goes on.

So I am extra thankful during this week of Thanksgiving to be getting out of here by tomorrow. We are so grateful that Chris's cousin offered to cook Thanksgiving dinner for our families this year. (otherwise we would have had Swanson Turkey TV dinners - of course I would have splurged for the selection of desserts to include the nutty chocolate brownie or cherry cobbler!) Most especially, I am so grateful that I get to go home and hug my family every night (and selfishly when they hug back I am really THANKFUL because there is a little less for them to hug!)

Please pray that you don't hear from me for a while because it means my life is uneventful. And to quote the awful late 70's TV with the most terrible actors, we are taking it *One Day at a Time.*

From: Marie Conley
Sent: Sun, Dec 2, 2012 4:24 pm
Subject: An important Evite

Ladies:

In a little bit, you will receive an evite to a very special party. When an adventure called Cushing's began June 13 and I started to share with you what an unusual journey I was about to embark on, you were all there cheering me on. Some of you were there from day one and some of you may have just joined, but in my eyes, there has been no difference. Your calls, e-mails, cards, notes, hugs, and tears strengthened my foundation and I was able to go on stronger each day!

If you are receiving this invitation, it is because somehow and in some way, YOU made an impact in my life. You have helped me get to this place, which is still not the finish line, but I am getting closer.

I have shared with many of you that I don't know how to begin to thank you and you then sweetly reply, "Please don't thank me."

So, this is NOT a thank you party. It's a "Come and hang with the girl" who has:

- A rare disease between two and ten people per million a year are diagnosed with

- A lunar adjective describing her chin

- A bison-like growth on her back

- A "twin" on the bottom of her foot (AKA the Chernobyl plantar wart that because of Cushing's has become my "mini me")

- An umbilical hernia (which the doctor attributed to childbirth even though I had my child six years before the diagnosis. That is still one of my favorites

- A weight gain of seventy plus pounds in twelve months (I will take credit and be happy for about four of those with cheese fries and nachos in that time frame - the rest just stinks - that's Cushing's)

- A recovering stress fracture in my hip

- One brain tumor - GONE

- Two adrenal glands - GONE

So let us celebrate all of these cool things. I am giving you ample notice.

Seriously, I appreciate how crazy your lives are but it would really mean a lot to me to have each of you in the same room so we can toast the true bond of friendship that has helped me live!

To my ladies who are in other states, I don't expect you to come but I needed you to know that you are part of my heart.

Love to you all and have a wonderful (and healthy) holiday!

From: Marie Conley
Sent: Sunday, December 02, 2012 9:05 PM
Subject: Home

Well at 4:45 pm, I sprang the joint! I am home and healthy (relatively speaking).

I have decided to call my two-night stay in the Penn State Hershey Hospital a **"Two-day getaway at a popular Hershey destination."** It sounds so much better.

No new news it's just part of the good old thing called Cushing's. If you recall, back in the day, when I shared some information about this disease, my doctor emphasized that this disease is very deceiving... surgeries are the easy part (it still makes me giggle that a six-hour brain surgery is easy!) The difficult part is the day after the successful surgery and the next 12 months!

Well, three hospital stays in less than six weeks I am a believer. We, as a family, have this nailed down. I know what floor I like to stay on and what nurses I hope to get. Carter knows to carry my medical records folder and to show Daddy where to get me a cup of tea (and a moose-track ice cream bar for himself) - it is all-good.

We could not do this without our family and friends pinch-hitting for us when this happens, so thank you!

As I said to my nurses today -- See ya' next time!

From: Marie Conley
Sent: Sunday, December 02, 2012 9:12 PM
Subject: Home – Correction

I should explain the last line - sorry.

I don't wish it to happen again. We are just realistic that we have some hurdles to still get through until my body adjusts to all of this.

As Coach Paterno said, "Think about getting up WHILE you're falling down."

Happy Holidays!

From: Marie Conley
Sent: Tuesday, December 04, 2012 8:33 PM
Subject: You couldn't make this up if you tried

So I knew I was a persuasive speaker but today I earned a medal. I had to go to Philly today for a follow-up appointment based on the last couple of weeks. My parents drove me down and I was planning to take the train back home. I wasn't feeling that great. As a standard, they had me get a blood check for sodium when I arrived. Long story short, I was starting to feel a little yucky while meeting with my nurse, Jayme, who was teaching me how to give myself my own injection of stress steroids. The blood work did not come while I was in the office - Jayme said she would phone me. Just like a TV show, as I was going to get a cab outside of the building, she called. I needed to come back up to the office as my sodium was 129 (remember, I need to be around 139-145 ---- the last two times I was admitted I was 122).

Long story long, rather than admitting me, Dr. Kharlip agreed (after I begged) to let me stay at my sister's house (a few blocks away). I have to monitor everything throughout the night. We are foregoing my DI medicine (AKA medicine that makes me stop peeing) and I will need to head back in tomorrow early for my blood tests. If I am good, they will monitor me for a couple hours and I go home. If not, I am admitted into University of Penn. Dr. Kharlip gave me her cell phone number and Christy and I can call if I start to tank and she will call me into the ER. I am their only patient with Cushing's disease and permanent DI so we are kind of experimenting here. HOWEVER, she does have a theory that seems to make sense. I will need to be patient, but I think it makes sense and can work.

Carter thinks I am having a girls' night at my sister's and that I will be home tomorrow.

PLEASE say a little prayer tonight. I do not want to go to back into the hospital, but if I do, I want it to be in Hershey.

I will keep you posted!

From: Marie Conley
Sent: Wednesday, December 5, 2012 5:02 PM
Subject: I'm home!

Your prayers worked. Thanks to my personal limo drivers Jean and Chuck Conley, I am home safe and sound. My counts are back up. I spent a lot of my time with my doctor and nurse and I think we have a good plan in place to avoid any immediate future ER visits. Last night was a little rough but it was NOT in the hospital. Again, my sister saves the day!

The next 72 hours are going to be a little tricky and uncomfortable and will require me to be close to home but I can still work, take care of my family, and get better, so all is good! SO... hopefully, no new drama e-mails from me for a while! Your prayers helped a ton. Who needs professional therapy when I have all of you?

Love you all!

From: Marie Conley
Sent: Saturday, December 22, 2012 3:14 PM
Subject: Things to be happy about

I am always writing about the not- so- great -things that are happening to me, so I wanted to share some good things -- my Top 10, if you will:

10. **My Belt** - Yes, I said belt. I now need a belt for a pair of jeans that I could barely put on after my surgery... and it needs the third hole!

9. **Fabiana and Laura** - My Cushing's Connections. They both have Cushing's disease and are in different stages of getting healthier. They are a true blessing for me.

8. **My parents** - Who listened to me cry on Monday because I didn't think I was going to have the energy this year to make crackle candy for Carter's teachers. All of the teachers made a big deal about this to him because they love the candy. My mom made four bags and my dad delivered them to me at the Reading exit of the Turnpike on Wednesday.

7. **My In-Laws** - For stepping in last Thursday and going to Carter's Christmas Play. I was stuck in the ER again. They and Chris cheered loudly for our little star!

6. **Nate, the masseuse** - I went to the Hotel Hershey Spa and had a hot stone massage. It was amazing and so relaxing. I did realize I am not ready yet as my buffalo hump does not like to be touched that way and it made it a little uncomfortable, BUT, nevertheless, it was magical.

5. **Strength** - I can beat my grandmother down the hallway now. I swear I could not do that two months ago. I am in PT and hangin' tough even if my bones are mush.

4. **Sophie Grace and Rosie** - They are the little British girls (my friends) on *The Ellen Show*. They have been my little source of strength since August. Every time I get sad, I YouTube them and all is right in the world. (I did actually e-mail Ellen to thank her for having Grace and Rosie on

her show, and told her my story. I want Ellen to have me on her show so I can let people know about Cushing's disease. Someone needs to get the word out, I will work on this later when I am healthier) For your viewing pleasure: http://www.youtube.com/watch?v=pP-PF4nKboI

3. **My Doctors** - This time last year I thought I was crazy and no one knew what was wrong with me and now I am on the road to recovery with a failed brain surgery, bi-lateral adrenalectomy and four hospital stays under my belt. (which is now on the third notch!)

2. **ONE WEEK** - Yesterday was the first time I have been one week free of blood tests and hospital stays: NOTHING since August 3rd!

1. **My family and friends** - Chris, Carter, and I would not have gotten this far without each and every one of you.

HAPPY HOLIDAYS, MERRY CHRISTMAS
and a HEALTHY New Year!

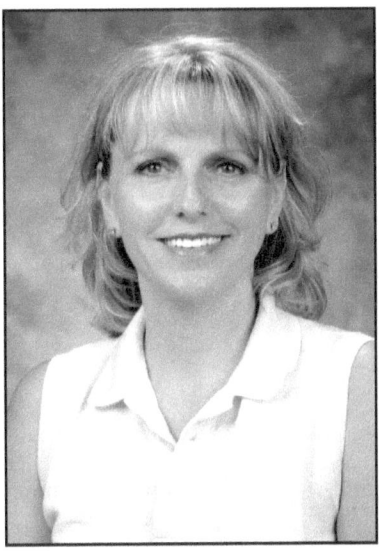

June 2009: Five months after this photo was taken, I started to experience bouts of bronitichis, pneumonia, strep, and shingles. Cushing's disease affects your immune system.

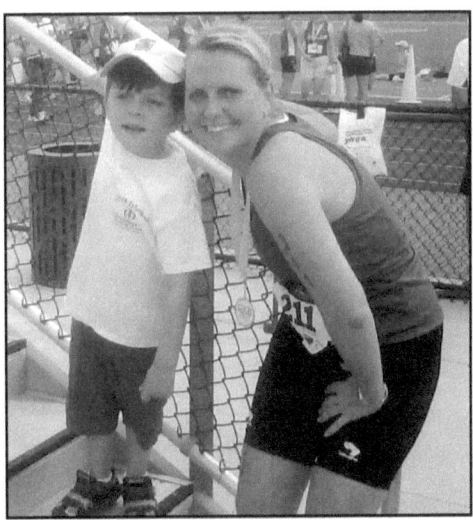

June 2010: Determined to compete in my first Sprint Triatholon. I barely crossed the finish line because little did I know I had a fractured right hip. I was on crutches for over three months and in PT for four months. Cushing's disease causes bone brittleness.

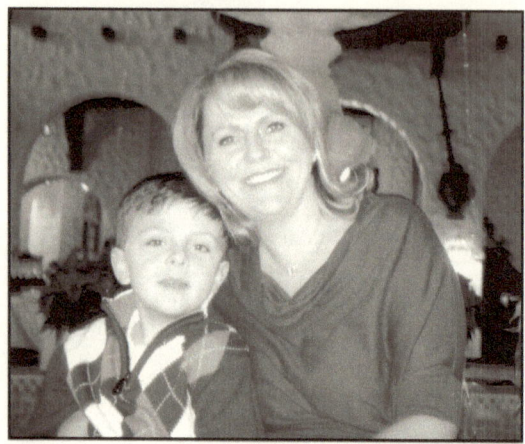

December 2011: I was gaining unexplained weight and could barely could sleep through the night. Cushing's disease affects your metabolism. Your body can not break down carbohydrates, proteins, and sugars properly. Cushing's patients have difficulty sleeping because their adrenal glands are producing too much cortisol. It felt like I did shots of espresso every night around 11 pm.

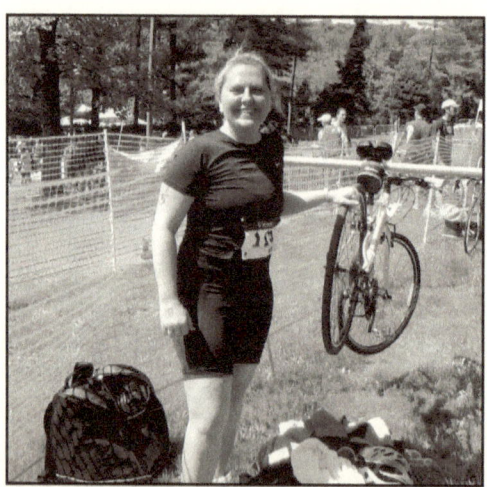

May 2012: I completed my second Sprint Triatholon. At this point, I had seen more than five specialists trying to figure out what was going on. No one could explain the weight gain – my face was so swollen and red all of the time. Five weeks later I was diagnosed with Cushing's disease. My doctor said my body was drowning in cortisol.

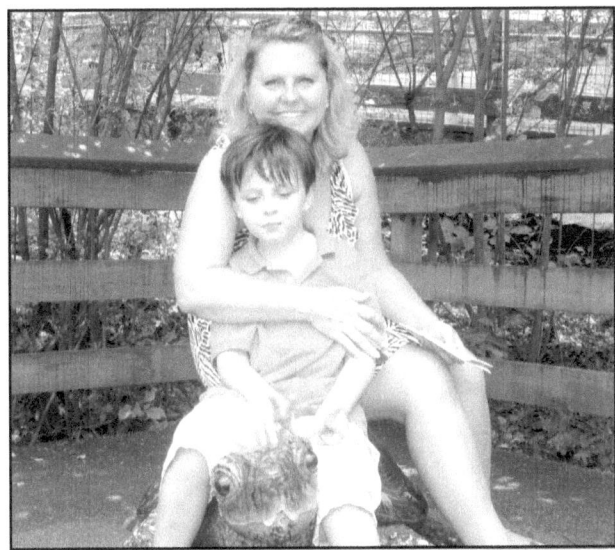

August 2012: Chris and I took Carter to the zoo before we told him that I would be in the hospital for of couple days because mommy had a boo-boo in her head. This picture was taken two weeks before my pitituary/brain surgery.

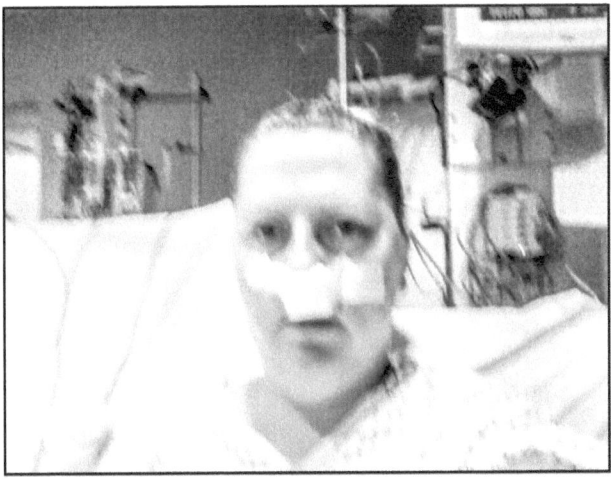

August 2012: The only thing I could do was laugh and take this pathetic "selfie." This "bandage" was used to catch possible cerebral leakage. My surgery was deemed medically unsuccessful. I had diabetes insipidus and was stuck in the IUC for ten days and I had this hidious bandaid. Awesome!

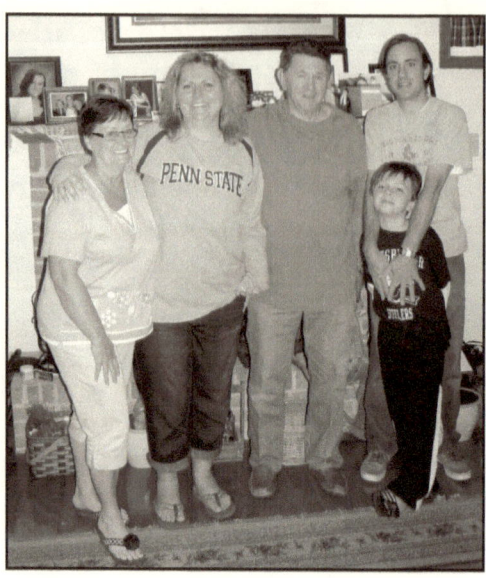

October 2012: We went to my in-laws the weekend before I was having my adrenals removed. This picture was taken the day before I went into the hospital. At this point, I had gained more than 20 pounds since May. I could barely walk up the steps or get off the couch and was having difficulty breathing.

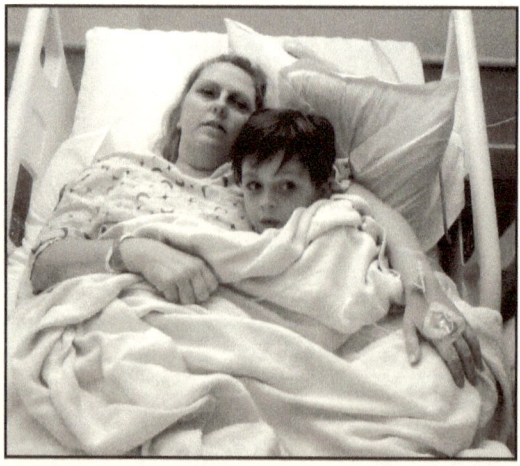

November 2012: For four months after my bilateral adrenalectomy, I was in and out of the ER and hospital six times. Chris, Carter and I made the best of it.

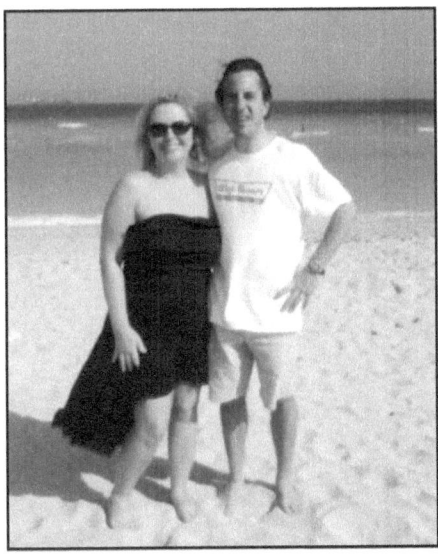

February 2013: We went to Miami to celebrate a friends birthday. I didn't make it past 9:00 pm any night but we were determined to kick Cushing's butt - better to do it in Miami then Hershey.

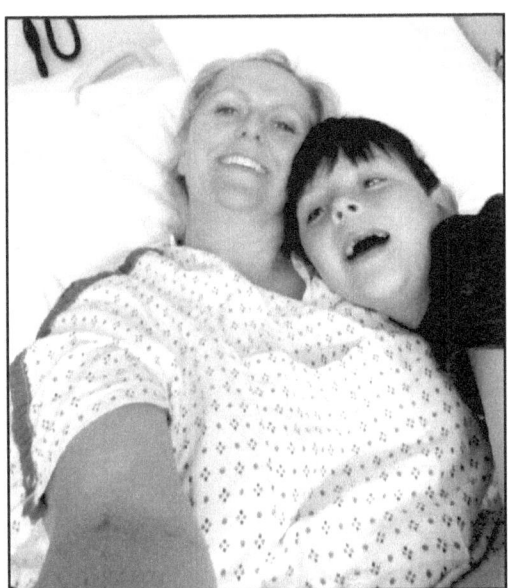

April 2013: One of my many stays at Penn State Hershey Medical Center for an adrenal crisis or low sodium due to my diabetes insipidus.

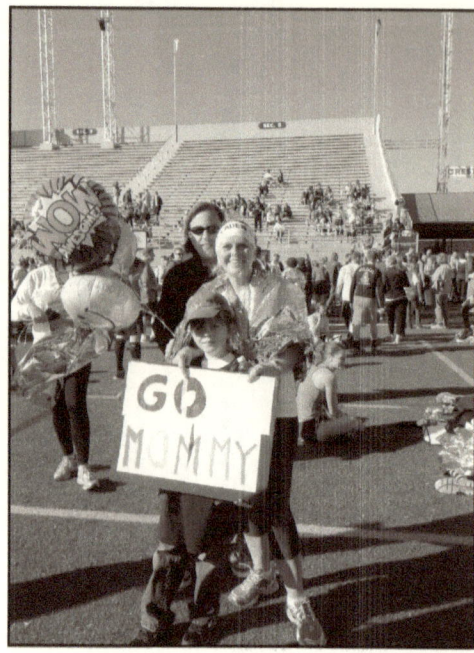

October 2013: With each email I wrote, I tried to end with the number of days leading up to the Hershey Half Marathon. I wasn't able to complete 13.1 but with the help of my friend, Cathy Boyle, we were a great relay team.

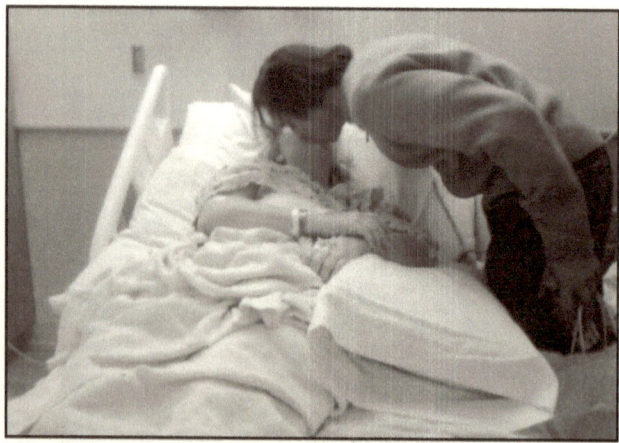

April 2014: This not having adrenals thing was getting old – an everyday occurance for one person can land me in the hospital. At least I was still getting kisses!

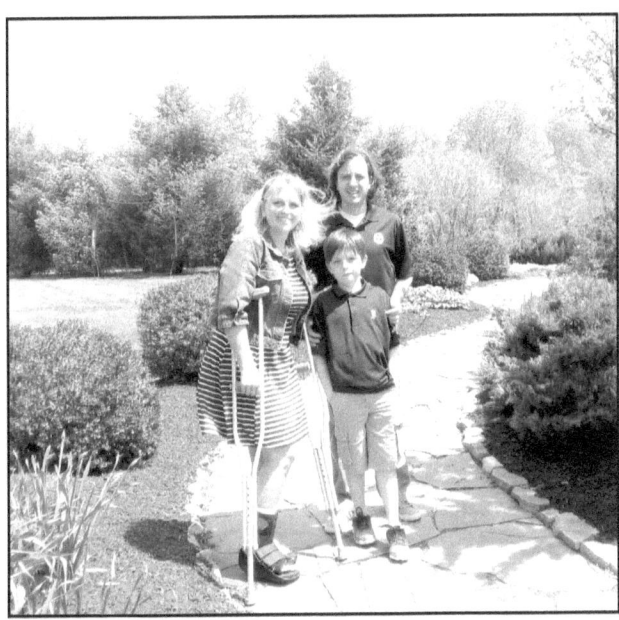

May 2014: While trying to showoff and catch a pitch from Carter, I fell and had a severe sprain. It landed me back in the hospital; was given a stress dose of steroids; and on crutches for two weeks!

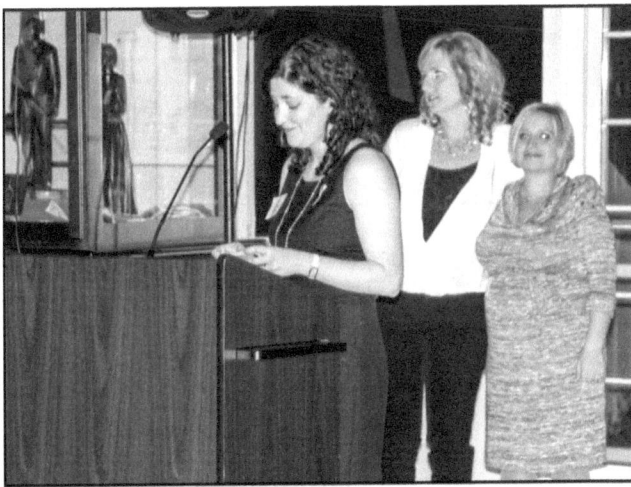

November 2014: Dr. Julia Kharlip, my endocrinologist and my "captain," spoke at The Kicking Cushing's to the Curb fundraiser and awareness reception. All funds raised supported The Conley Cushing's Disease Fund.

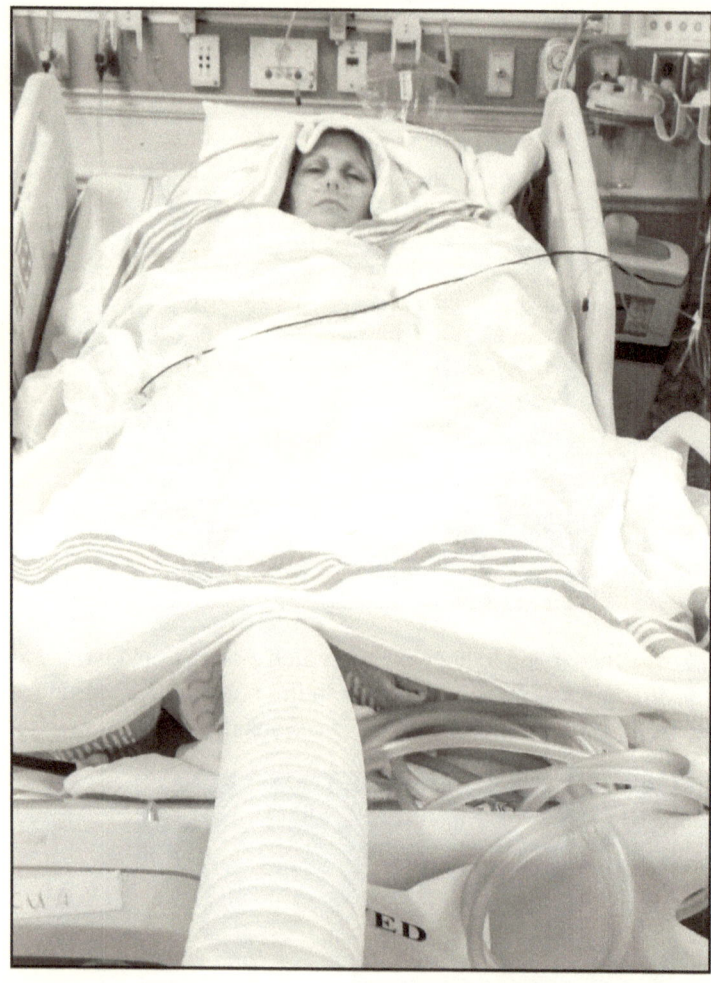

January 2015: I had a lower right lung resection at the Hospital of University of Pennsylvania in search of ACTH hormone.

Author's note: After my Cushing's Celebration in January

From: Marie Conley
Sent: Wednesday, January 16, 2013 10:50 PM
Subject: Post Cushing Debriefing

What a night! I cannot thank you enough for coming on Saturday. For those who could not attend, please know you were there in spirit. It meant so much to me that the people who will forever be in my heart for helping us through this were all in one room (or on this e-mail). It seems like everyone had a great time (and my recycling can supports this statement).

You all know I am not generally this "women only" kind of person but it was so amazingly appropriate for Saturday night. A couple of times, I just took a minute to take it all in. In one room, at the same time, there were women from all walks of life with so many different unique strengths and beautiful qualities. I have gained some sense of power, inspiration, humor, and humility from each of you. It is funny how differently I look at everything now.

I received some wonderful gifts, but during the chaos of the evening, I misplaced some cards. For those who brought a special little something, please know how appreciative I am and how it was completely unnecessary.

What kills me is that I have not had a chance to write personal thank you notes yet. I could come up with a thousand excuses of why I haven't, like:

- I have had a terrible reaction to my step-down since Monday

- have to get blood work to test a possible thyroid problem

- go back and forth to schedule my next surgery (March 28th - Holy Thursday). They say it should be a two-day stay!

- Work with my endocrinologist and attorney to prevent me from having to travel to Pittsburgh next week - I was subpoenaed to testify in an upcoming trial

- Schedule a MOHS procedure on my forehead (my doc says "better safe than sorry") and have a little section removed - cool... "Moon Face," "Buffalo Hump," now a Frankenstein-like scar on the side of my forehead that is not where my bangs lie!

- Oh yeah, be a mom, a wife and a professional

- and the VERY real excuse: I realized I ran out of my personal stationery!

So please accept this e-mail as a temporary thank you.

Please remember to use the Cushing's Cup (for those who could not attend, I will be sending yours in the mail). I admit to having a hidden agenda for the cups. What happens if you are using it and someone asks "What the heck is Cushing's disease?" Now you can tell them, I know this girl who was basically a red-hot mess; she had a "Moon Face," a "Buffalo Hump" and those are the nice things.

Seriously, what happens if someday you end up meeting, some-one who knows someone who has been sick and no one can figure it out and they have some of my symptoms... you might be able to tell them, you aren't sure but you might want them to talk to their doctors about Cushing's disease! You might be able to help diagnose someone and help save his or her life.

For those who have asked that this become an annual event....
this is not a bad idea.

*Author's note: All guests toasted to kicking Cushing's with a glass
that said "My friend has Cushing's disease and all I got was this
stinkin' cup!"*

From: Marie Conley
Sent: Sunday, February 24, 2013 9:54 PM
Subject: Thank you

Sister and Mrs. Mussoline, {*Carter's principal and second grade
teacher*}

Thank you so much for allowing Carter to miss a week of school
to go on a vacation. I would like to share that he experienced
educational outings every day but he did not. What he did experience was a time with his family without one trip to the ER.
Equally important, my parents and Chris laughed and smiled
and did not have a worried look (often) on their faces for almost
six days in a row.

I took a picture of Carter and me while we were on the beach rid-
ing bikes. It was amazing. My doctors and Physical Therapists
would have killed me, but for three days in a row, Carter and I
rode our bikes on the sand. I took the picture right after he said
to me, "Mommy, I'm glad you got your muscles back." I was reminded hourly that I was still not better and I could not join my
family for many activities, but that was truly OK. I spent four
hours in the doctor's office today and have two ear infections, a
sinus infection, and an upper respiratory infection, but our bike
rides on the beach were worth it. We respect and value Carter's
education and did not take it lightly that he would miss five days

of school, but he needed it. He did all of his assignments and hopefully is caught up.

Again, Chris and I cannot thank you enough.

From: Marie Conley
Sent: Monday, February 25, 2013 11:47 PM
Subject: Cushing's Phase II- The Crappy Part

Sorry this is long.

Dear friends,

I have been meaning to write this for some time. I have not seen, spoken to and sometimes not responded to many of you for about six weeks. I feel terrible that I have not been a good friend or a good family member. I appreciate your patience and, as always, your e-mails and texts mean the world to me.

I have been trying to figure out what the heck has been going on and more importantly, how to articulate it. Unfortunately, the only person who understands my "language" is Fabiana, my Cushing's partner- in -crime. I am certainly not giving up or giving in, but I am, for the first time, acknowledging, that I am actually sick. I am reminded of this hourly. The irony is my physical appearance is slowly changing (I hope for the better). I have cheekbones and I believe I saw a rib when I was dashing by the mirror the other day.

I completely have accepted that I am in **Phase II- the crappy part**! A hole in my brain, eight holes in my stomach, 10 crappy days in the ICU, permanent kidney damage, a "Buffalo Hump," a freaky-ass hernia (soon to be fixed March 27th), taking meds four times a day, PT twice a week, a nutritionist twice a week and eight visits to the ER since October – that is easy! I can handle that. There was a diagnosis; we came up with a plan - if detoured, we rerouted, went back on course and moved on to implement a plan to get me healthy.

This is the crazy part the doctor warned me about when first diagnosed in June. This is what Fabiana said could happen when we spoke in August (she is six months ahead of me in recovery). There is really no easy way to explain this but I will try so you understand my challenges right now. While this aspect is temporary and I know in my head it will work itself out within the next six months, it is unfortunately real and candidly, hell.

OK, I pretend I have about 20 points a day. Each thing I do – I mean mentally and physically – gets points. Once my points are done – I am done! Therefore, every Sunday, I need to look at my week and try to figure out what gets my points daily. (Editor's note: This is my way of explaining it and has NO medical rationale attached to it). The basics: Getting Carter ready for school – 2 points (that is assuming there are no freak-outs). Showering and getting ready for my day – 2 points. Intense meetings anywhere from 5 to 10 points. Running Carter to games and practices – 5 points. PT – 5 points. Work prep for meetings, research, calls -5 points; doing household chores – 2 points; ----- I think you get the point. This is with the understanding that I KNOW everything that will happen. Any surprises or additional stress takes points away. I then have to figure out which upcoming activities will require more points. I have to be careful the night before and morning after.

For those of you who have known me for more than a minute, you know I love working and being active. For good or bad, right or wrong, I love it. It has been, and is, my safe haven. This disease is now robbing me of this. I accepted not running and working out (for now). But working, heck, I was creating an access database the day after my brain surgery. I was on a State System conference call from my hospital room the day after the bi-lateral adrenalectomy. This part is just BS.

This really stinks. There are days that the thought of reading an e-mail or doing the seven dishes in the sink, could literally knock me out. So, this is a very long way of asking all of you to please be patient with me. I know I will get through this next phase but right now, my body and my brain chemical makeup are challenging every aspect of my livelihood. I am so lucky to have Chris, an amazing partner, and Carter, who is my little buddy and helper. My parents and in-laws always offer to help but as shocking as this may be, I hate asking for help! I am very involved with my Board work for the State System. I love my work with the Paterno family and have taken a new role in assisting Sue with creating a pilot program with a national group, Stop It Now! to create awareness and prevention of child sexual abuse on college campuses. (On a side note, I have never met a more compassionate family: supporting me professionally while caring for me personally). And I work with my dearest friend, Lauren, who allows my creative juices to flow but is like my mother and cuts me off if I am doing too much. I think all of this work sometimes actually makes me feel like I am getting points back.

Please understand this is not a pity party. (There would have been many more curses.) I am just trying to let those who mean the most to me, and those who have traveled this road with me, in on my little secret.... Shhhhhh, I guess I am sick!

Once I am better, Fabiana and I will work on creating ways to drive awareness to this disease. We have spoken about a study on the "brain fogginess" part (this drives the two of us crazy) but we were told we don't have a large sampling to be funded. I am going to step up my efforts to get on the "Ellen" show. What better platform to bring about awareness of this disease while laughing at my "Buffalo Hump?"

For now, I plot and dream every night of crossing that finish line in October at the Hershey Half.

I miss you all. And please know that you mean so much to me that this e-mail took a good 5 points to compose and edit!

From: Lauren Cotter Brobson
Sent: Thursday, March 28, 2013 9:58 PM
Subject: Marie's Surgery Went Well

To all of Marie's Ladies:

I do not have many details, but Marie (via Chris) has asked that I let you all know that her hernia surgery went well — even better than expected. She is in pain, but at the very least, they were able to make the repair, which really did need to be made. I suspect she is cranky because they got off to a late start and she, of course, couldn't eat or drink beforehand, and she wasn't settled into her hospital room until around 7 pm this evening. We all know, however, that she is in good hands at University of Penn. Please keep her in your thoughts and prayers (along with Chris and Carter, too) as she begins yet again, another road to recovery. I am sure you will all be hearing from her with more details and her customary good-humored commentary very soon.

Author note: E-mail was printed with the permission of Lauren Cotter Brosbon, a close family friend.

From: Marie Conley
Sent: Saturday, March 30, 2013 2:26 PM
Subject: Three is a charm

Hey all. I got to my parents' place last night and will be here through Monday. All is good. The surgery went well. Carter had the best time with his Aunt Christy in the city. I need to be careful for the next two weeks (no driving) and will have to avoid lifting anything over three pounds for the next six to eight weeks. My parents are coming up and taking shifts this week and next so we are very lucky to have that support in place. I have great pain meds and antibiotics and will have enough steroids in me for the next five days so I won't feel a thing if I am attacked by a huge germ. Because of all of the stress steroids, I could pick up a house and crush it! The great news is I am done. It will be a pain in the butt for the next couple of weeks but I will be able to begin PT in six weeks and start to train again for races (and life) soon.

I will continue to focus on getting better, being patient, and adjusting to being the square peg that needs to fit into a round hole for the next six months or so until my body and my medicines align. As Dr. Kharlip reminds me, it will take about a year. She explained that due to Cushing's, every tissue in my body needs to learn how to function again. It doesn't happen at once; it just happens. Being adrenal insufficient and having the permanent DI (kidney/sodium thing) will become much more manageable once all of the other stuff shakes out! I continue to remind myself that in the scheme of things I am still so very lucky. I experimented yesterday and tried something new in the hospital. My doctors do rounds by 6:00 am so I snuck into the bathroom (which is a little tricky when you are hardwired to monitors and oxygen, but I am a pro by now) by 5:30 am and fixed my hair and did my makeup so when they came in, I looked better than my labs would tell them. One of the residents said, "She has color in her cheeks and looks good." Little did he know that it was Chanel bronzing powder! I spoke with my doctors later that morning and because I know how I felt, they discharged me knowing that I was only thirty minutes from the hospital; I am enjoying not being in a hospital bed.

I am the lucky one who gets to come home and decorate Easter eggs with my son and husband!

Chris and I cannot thank you enough for your prayers, humor, and support. It has been a long journey since June of last year, but we truly believe the worst is behind us and the best is yet to come!

Happy Easter and see you all soon.

From: Marie Conley
Sent: Monday, June 03, 2013 1:51 AM
Subject: Friends

I am not quite sure how to begin this and a lot of me doesn't even want to write it. The wonderful people on here can help me through the next week in a couple of different ways... some with Carter, some with the house, some with the dogs (we have my parents' crazy fourteen month-old puppy right now), some with Carter and baseball, and all of you with me if I lose it - so far I am good!)

Two weeks ago, on Monday, I was in a fender bender -- a pretty decent jab from behind was enough to scare the crap outta' me. I went to the ER to get my stress dose of steroids, but more importantly, to make sure my belly was OK since I just had surgery seven weeks before. The good news is everything in my belly looked good --- my right outside lung - not so much. My girl,

Sheilah, was in the ER at Penn State Hershey waiting for me –she rocks. I think that is why I got a good robe.

I am not going to get into all of the medical stuff because I don't know much. I know enough to know that last Tuesday, I was down at University of Penn to see a lung doctor per my endocrinologist and my primary here. The doctor I saw was wonderful and knows enough about my history so I am back at Penn in the hospital all day Wednesday and Thursday this week for tests. Chris and I will then go down to meet with a lung specialist on Friday.

I hope we find out something on Friday, but unfortunately, we probably will not know much. The doctors went to the dark side and said the words that I clearly thought were forbidden on all of my medical forms - UNUSUAL or RARE. My problem is that the placement of this nodule is UNUSUAL and it cannot be biopsied without surgery (at least that is what a group of them have already said).

I don't have fancy medical words to look up this time or anything. I have hours of scans and dyes on Wednesday and Thursday (I think this is to rule certain things out) and our first real meeting is on Friday. There doesn't seem to be any initial thought that this is from Cushing's disease. I had a chest scan in July before my first surgery and they saw "something" that they dismissed as a mucus impaction. Well, it has grown slightly and it is VERY unlikely this is what this is.

We chose not to share this with my parents or any family (other than my sister) as they are on a great vacation and will be back on Thursday. They should enjoy themselves - they worked their whole lives to have these trips. While I missed my mommy, she and my dad would have cancelled the rest of their vacation and drove straight back home. Honestly for what? I will wake up tomorrow, make pancakes for Carter, and move through our day as planned.

With the guidance and counsel of Carter's play therapist, Jamie, we told Carter what was happening. We have learned that when we try to hide something, he picks up on it. He said he was used to it. It wasn't mean: just a matter of fact. In retrospect, our timing was probably bad. The Red Sox/Yankees were on TV (now that is the tragedy. My son does not know who he likes more: the Yanks or Red Sox... (My Tastycake, cheesesteak, Yo-yelling soul is dying!) Chris is remarkable. We don't have many facts to check, so it is all about just waiting until we know what to do next.

So here I am asking for a couple things, if I may be so bold... prayers - more for Chris and Carter and honestly my parents (when I tell them). Thanks in advance - to the many friends helping with Carter this week. Should I need a quick backup I know I can call on any one of you. Fortunately, he is scheduled for "Camp Babci" and Pop-Pop all next week, so that will help if I need to go back and forth to the hospital. It might be a little while until we find out what this little bugger is, but between now and then, if you could give God a little shout-out for me that would be great. I will keep you posted... as we explained to Carter, we are not worrying about it. I placed it in the "worry box." We put our worry thoughts in a box. We would take them back out when we had to – if we don't have to worry about them – we will throw them away. We will bring it out if and when we have to but for now, it is in the box.

From: Marie Conley
Sent: Saturday, June 08, 2013 12:21 AM
Subject: Update

Hey all. I am so sorry for not getting back sooner. While I am not trying to make excuses, it has been a very long 17 days since the accident and a very long 72 hours of appointments. I will cut to the chase: no news is good news (at least that is how we are spinning it). So what does that mean? The tests this week were long, uncomfortable, and intimidating. As expected, the Octreoscans done on Wednesday and Thursday did not show anything, meaning they confirmed the cells were not carcinoid cells, which are specific types of cancer cells. That was great news.

The "bugger" (as I will call it) was confirmed to be in a very weird place. As I explained, it cannot be accessed through a scope or biopsied through a needle biopsy. To make matters more interesting, the bugger is on my right lung near the diaphragm. What this means is that every time I breathe and they try to capture a picture, it will never be the same picture, never look the same. (Really, does this surprise anyone?) So we are not quite sure if it has grown in the past year or hasn't. I have homework to do, and that is to try to see if there were any films taken of my abdomen before July 2012 to see if it was there before.

Dr. Pechet, the thoracic surgeon at the University of Penn, can't say with hundred percent certainty that it is nothing to worry about, BUT given what he can see, at this time, it does not have the shape of something he would be immediately concerned with. The only real option for certainty is to have it surgically removed and biopsied.

To ensure we understood all options, we discussed the surgery. We must remember one thing - let's call this the backdrop - as it pertains to my "insides"... I have lots going on between the Cushing's disease thing, the sodium/DI thing, and the adrenal thing. I am not the strongest, medically. Here is the low-down on what would have to happen. They put me out and remove the tumor (laparoscopically) going through my ribs. I would be in the hospital for a day or two. During my stay, they would insert some kind of epidural thing into my back that would remain for a couple of weeks to ensure that I am coughing all of the time and moving around so I don't get pneumonia.

Now, having not spoken at all to my captain, Dr. Kharlip, I know enough about my disease and its little friends that this surgery would mean I would have to be on a much higher dose of my steroids for a longer time while this is going on. Clearly, I would have to stop running my 10 miles a day (just kidding, wanted to see if you were still reading) and honestly, I do not have the best luck with hospitals! Dr. Pechet wants us to weigh all of the potential risks against the benefits at this time. Things I need to think about: going through my ribs -- are my bones strong enough now that one wouldn't crack during the procedure? Am I ready to have large doses of steroids, then taper down again? Do I want to be out of commission for a couple of weeks? And, I am sure there are more questions we would have to weigh.

Dr. Pechet was honest, and concise. I am going to work on finding any films that may exist at Penn State, and am scheduled for another CT scan of my chest in October. At that time, we will have another discussion with him. He explained to Chris and me, even if I did not have all of this other stuff going on and I exhibited all of the same signs I am showing now, he would say wait.

Earlier in the week, I spoke with a person, whom I trust and respect. He was kind enough to share an experience similar to mine. Having this knowledge helped me get through this week. I have seen him since his surgery and I understand that there is a "wait and see" period before the surgery and he is stronger and better than ever.

So, we wait. That is where we are.

I have lost two summers to this disease: last year, waiting for the brain surgery and limited in almost every way and the summer before spent on crutches with my fractured hip. Chris and Carter deserve a wife and mother who can do things, like walk and run, and ride roller coasters and play on the beach! I would love to have more certainty but, sick or not sick, who would not! I trust my doctors. I have had more blood tests and checks than most humans have. I am more in tune to my body than I ever thought I would be. If I have a copper taste in my mouth - like pennies - then I need to adjust one medicine. If the taste in my mouth is more like another metal, then I have to adjust another medicine. One type of headache means one thing over another type. I am totally cool with that - it is my new normal but I am also cool with not adding something else onto my plate for the next couple of months knowing that no real damage will be done!

There are no words to express how grateful Chris and I are for all you have done. Thank you so much - all of you - for your prayers and help over these past two weeks. I don't know how Chris and I would have done it without you. So many of you helped care for Carter that he didn't miss a game or practice or school function. He has been a champ through all of it. Chris, as always, is a pillar of strength and humor. Thank you to everyone who helped take care of my parents' crazy puppy while he was here. We were able to avoid telling my parents about the "bugger" in my lung- they get back from their vacation tonight and will be coming up here tomorrow. We will talk to them at that time.

So, here's to trying to get back to the regular things: getting stronger by going to PT, dropping this *#^@$^@* weight, working, living, and negotiating with Carter why he can't stay up to 10:00 pm and just because he is a third grader now and why he can't use "bad" words.

So here's to a great summer.

PS: The most important thing... Chris got a hole-in-one yesterday at a golf outing at the Hershey Links and won a two-year free lease on a Lincoln. How cool is that!

From: Marie Conley
Sent: Tuesday, October 08, 2013 3:58 PM
Subject: One year

As I was looking at the calendar last week making sure I knew what day Carter has hockey or soccer and ensuring I have all of my professional deadlines locked in and what I was going to make for dinner, I kept thinking something was weird about the date October 8. It was one year ago today that I parted with my two dear friends, adrenal 1 and adrenal 2. While they were two little bitty glands, they left a tremendous hole in my body and soul!

I am sharing this with a small few, who have stayed by my side through e-mails and calls: some of whom I have clung to and others I may have unintentionally pushed away. To the ones who mean the most, I wanted to share with you some information given to me as I have been searching for some answers. It is a lot and I am not expecting you to read it all but I pulled out some of the pieces that spoke to me and what I have gone through and continue to go through on a daily basis.

To the ones who know me best, I tried not to inconvenience anyone. I tried to be strong and not be a typical "Cushing's patient, and it seems like, in the end, I am exactly like a "Cushing's patient" and the only difference is now I am starting to be OK with that. I have made many mistakes, but never intentionally, and sometimes while I was truly in a survival mode. I never meant to hurt anyone and I know that sometimes I did. My journey is not a typical one and that is OK, too! Between the brain surgery, adrenal surgery, and hernia, and in addition to the ER and hospital stays, I have been in University of Penn or Penn State Hershey thirteen times since last August. **But** since July, I have taught Carter to dive into the lake in NH at my Aunt Linda and Uncle Joe's lake house, and as a family we went biking almost every day down the shore, and we ran a 5K race on Sunday preparing for my Hershey Half Marathon next Sunday (RELAY with my buddy Cathy). Carter, Chris, and I have figured out how to deal with this on a daily basis and we are doing fine.

A friend suggested I keep a journal and in a way, as I look back, my e-mails to you have been just that, my journal to help share what I clearly cannot articulate.

I leave on Thursday for another round of tests and meet with the doctors again on Friday regarding the spot on my lung. My mom is going to the doctor's appointments with me. I will keep you informed as to what the doctor says and what we will decide to do. Just say a prayer for me!

From: Marie Conley
Sent: Friday, October 11, 2013 5:13 PM
Subject: Can't touch this...

I just wanted to drop a quick note to say --- no surgery. The scans continue to show a growth but without getting into too many crazy medical details, the doctors saw that there were calcium spots in the growth... probably due to all of the bouts of pneumonia and bronchitis...probably scar tissue...yadda yadda yadda... no surgery - no worries. They will monitor "the bugger" but it is off my radar screen. All of my other stuff is all Cushing's related and that is just life and that is fine with me. We are so happy. Thank you so much for your prayers and thoughts!

Nine days from now - I will have crossed the finish line at the Hershey Half!

Have a great weekend.

PS: We are going out and I am eating me some nachos!!!!!

From: Marie Conley
Sent: Monday, October 21, 2013 1:49 PM
Subject: I did it

It was ugly to watch but I did it! One of my best girls, Cathy, and I ran a relay for the Hershey Half yesterday. I ran 6.4 miles and crossed the finish line. Thank you so much for always cheering me on!

PS: The headband says "Caden" - I ran for one of the many special miracle kids at Penn State Hershey Children's Hospital.

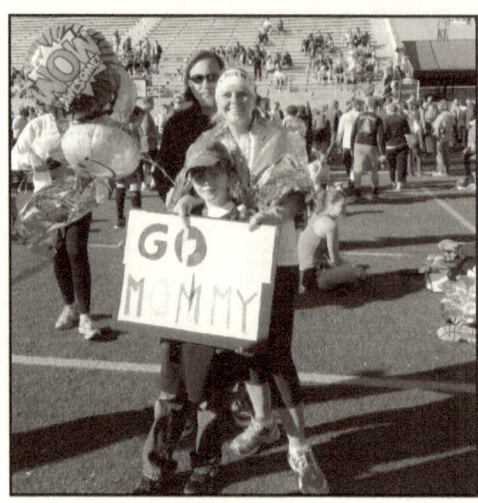

From: Marie Conley
Sent: Sunday, October 20, 2013 8:44 PM
To: My doctors (endocrinologist, neurologist, surgeons) PT specialists, my PA, my Reiki therapist
Subject: Thank you, Mr. Cushing's!

I just wanted to thank all of you for your help in getting me to this point. I will never be able to articulate the level of gratitude and appreciation I have for each one of you. While I still have a long way to go, I feel like I could not fully celebrate today without you. Some of you fixed my brain, others took my glands, some helped my bones, and others are obsessed with my output and sodium (just kidding!). If you are on this list, it is because you always cared for my family and me. Every e-mail I sent out to friends and family, since I was diagnosed last June with Cushing's disease, whether it was about the brain surgery, removal of my adrenal glands, hernia surgery, hospital stays or 10 ER visits - concluded with a countdown about the Hershey Half Marathon and my goal to cross the finish line. As the former director of the Children's Miracle Network (the benefactor of this race) and as part of its inaugural planning committee of the event with a great crew from the Hershey Entertainment & Resorts Co. and a finisher in 2009, the Hershey Half has always meant so much to me. Today, the race had an entirely different meaning as I crossed the finish line as part of a relay team. For the first time in almost two years, I felt, for the 6.4 miles I ran, like the old Marie Conley. While saving lives is truly part of your job descriptions, I hope you know that you saved mine in so many ways.

PS: Dr. Kharlip, can you please share this with Drs. Sirisena and Sawan as I owe a huge thank you to them as well.

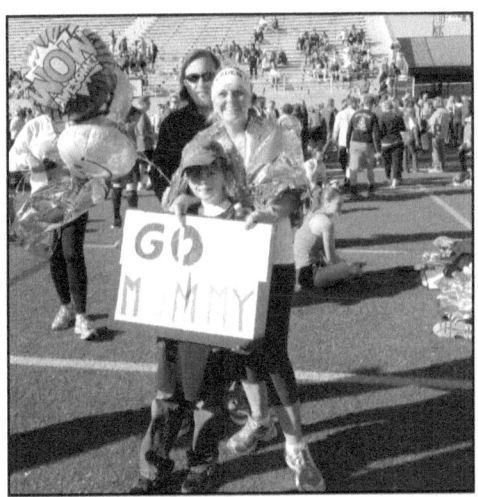

From: Marie Conley
Sent: Sunday, April 06, 2014 4:28 PM
Subject: A funny pain in the butt update

I hope this e-mail finds you well. It has been a while since I have e-mailed my core group of peeps with any updates --- my current experience compels me to write. As you all know, I have been doing my best to just keep moving forward. For some on this e-mail, it has been a while since I have seen you, but I am always thinking of my friends and family and how lucky I am. I continue to learn to balance and allot "my daily 20 points" the best I can, giving Carter whatever he needs, then filling in the rest professionally and personally. Some weeks I have many points to spare, and other weeks, it is all I can do to get through the day.

It has been a great couple of months! Carter is doing very well and growing like a weed. I have continued to work well and smartly and believe that the work I am doing with the Paterno family will truly have an impact in helping to make significant changes in the world of child sexual abuse prevention and awareness. I continue to exercise to get stronger and will not accept that I cannot be the size I once was. Chris continues to be a pillar of strength and laughter.

Some may not know that I was able to get a second opinion at the University of Virginia with two of the country's top leading doctors in the Cushing's world in January. They agreed that the care I am receiving at the University of Penn (love Dr. Kharlip and her team) is excellent. They reinforced (rather stressed) to my mom and me that my complication with the Diabetes Insipidus (my kidney messaging thingie) and my lack of adrenal glands make this combination a very serious and medically challenging illness to manage and there is really nothing more anyone can do!!! (Always good to have a cold wet slap to the face of reality with a touch of Southern hospitality.)

I went to the Cushing's Support and Research Foundation conference in Atlanta at the end of February. It was very interesting and I appreciated the opportunity to listen as a spectator rather than a patient in my doctor's office. It was also surreal being in a room with a group of individuals who, without saying a word, understand what I was going through. Most especially, it made me realize how very lucky I am. I will be working on setting up a support group for Cushing's patients in the Central PA, Philadelphia and tristate area. Fabiana will be helping me with the one in Philly. There are surprisingly about 70 some people in the area on all different spectrums of the disease. Who knows how many will embrace the opportunity? I believe it would be a nice resource for us to meet a couple of times a year.

Since all of you on this e-mail have experienced this journey with me (us), through tears and laughter, I felt I was robbing you of a great experience. I know full well that, as I share this, I will be living through the humiliation again. I am also aware that for most on this e-mail I will be providing you so much future ammunition for jokes....

We all know this journey has come with its share of embarrassing tales...speaking of tails...

On Friday morning, I started to experience some pain in my bottom region. I will not go any further but to share that while I was pregnant with Carter I experienced a similar problem (and for only a few - I will just say duct tape). Anyway, the pain progressed.

My parents and Babci (Polish for grandmother) were on the way up to our house because Carter was playing "Jesus" in the living stations on Friday afternoon at school. We were meeting Chris's mom and Aunt Shirley at church to watch Carter's performance and then we were all going to meet up later for dinner at our house. So,...I am not enjoying sitting on a wooden pew at church and Chris insists that I call my PA, Michael Fedor (who is my guardian angel) to have him take a look because we know from experiences that this could get serious quickly. I see Michael at 3:50 pm and by 4:45 pm my mom and I were in the ER. Chris joined me at the ER and my mom went back to the house with

Carter. The specialist (whose specialty rhymes with mocktologist) explains the procedure, which includes a local anesthetic (yes boys and girls multiple needles...). I will share that I would have rather had another hole drilled through my cranium then ever have this done again AWAKE!!! It was not pleasant, but at least the doctor had a sense of humor because the only way to save myself in such a "vulnerable" position was to joke about it. Chris often shared that he would like to start doing something different, like "go out" on Friday nights. I believe I fulfilled his wish with a new type of Friday night experience. I can only imagine what his version of this story will be when he retells it with a couple of beers in him, as I would not let him leave the room. I went home by 11:00 pm and landed back in the hospital by 8:30 am the next morning. Even though the mocktologist consulted with my team down at University of Penn and I was given more meds to counterbalance not having adrenal glands, the pain management component put my Cushing's stuff into a quick downward spiral. I could not keep anything down which immediately put me back into the hospital.

So, I write this while in my hospital bed awaiting to be discharged sometime tonight, hopefully, in time to see some of Carter's baseball game at 6:00 pm. I will need to take it easy over the next couple of days, top to bottom (ha ha), while my body tapers off all of the hydrocortisone that has gone into me over the last 72 hours. Again, perhaps you feel I shared too much, but for most of you on this e-mail, I would be robbing you of such an unbelievably unusual (yet so typical) experience for me on this great journey of health!

Enjoy and can't wait to see you soon.

From: Marie Conley
Sent: Friday, November 14, 2014 7:56 AM - *Morning of the First Annual Kickin' Cushing's to the Curb fundraiser for The Conley Cushing's Disease Fund.*
Subject: Thank you

By the time you get this, I will be long gone to bed (I preset the e-mail). I just wanted to thank you all for your help and support throughout the past several months. I am very excited about tomorrow and crazy nervous but most of you will be in the crowd so I will look at you all for strength (or a little giggle). I will probably be very overwhelmed and be spread pretty thin so in case I don't fully show my appreciation and gratitude, I wanted to do it now. While you may not have thought you did much, knowing you were all behind me gave me the strength in these last couple of months that I truly needed. I look forward to seeing some of you around 11:30 am tomorrow at the Hall. Good news today was What If and Purcell Hall laid everything down with linens, so less for us to do tomorrow -yeah! If anyone sticks around until the end (and you all better) - if you can lend a hand to go through whatever is left on the tables onto the registration desk - I would appreciate it. What If is going to take care of most of it but I still need more help.

I am attaching the new website that my friend Karen designed -- it is simple for the time being but the donation key is active and I am going to post it tomorrow on Facebook and Twitter. I am also attaching my logo if you want to post it on your Facebook pages.

Thank you again for your support, but most importantly your friendship.

Author's note: Sent to a very small group of friends.

From: Marie Conley
Sent: Monday, December 29, 2014 11:11 PM
Subject: Greetings

Friends:

I hope you had a great Christmas/holiday. We had a wonderful time with our families. Over the last two weeks and subsequent weeks leading up to them, I have been struggling a bit and have gone underground like I normally do when I feel like this (not returning calls, cancelling social things, hunkering down). I am attempting to pull myself out a little bit and realize that many times in the past when I felt like this, I would e-mail you all. Maybe it was because I was getting it out of my head and onto paper; maybe it was sharing the information with people who mean the most; maybe it is about not feeling alone; or maybe it is because it is easier for me to sometimes hide behind this laptop, but regardless I always felt better and at peace.

Since June 2013 (as you know), I have seen a pulmonologist five times in addition to my endocrinologist because they found that "thingie" on my right lung. The main problem, and why he has to monitor this so often, is because they cannot do a biopsy. It is located in such a funky spot - near the bottom of my right lung but very close to my diaphragm - they can't really get in there to get a sample (the whole breathing thing is getting in the doctor's way). After seeing one pulmonologist, I saw my current doctor/surgeon; we have been on a roller coaster. First it was, "It probably isn't anything, let's see you back in six months." In July, he said, "Well, that's odd...it grew, but the percentage was really low" and two weeks ago, we (Chris and Mom) are where I am now in a "black hole."

On one hand, they don't think it is growing like a malignant tumor would grow and threw out some percentages that it may be less than ten percent this, or three percent that or yada yada yada. On Dec. 19, Dr. Kharlip came to the mindset that I have had ---- let's get it out. I truly, deep in my bones and gut, believe that this is where the Cushing's cells are and that it needs to come out. (When they did the tissue biopsy of the pituitary tumor and the adrenal tissue - the Cushing's (ACTH cells) were not in there - there could still be cells left somewhere on the pituitary stalk or in my sinus cavity but we will never know). If these are ACTH cells - they have a very high percentage of becoming cancerous when they are in the lungs - this form of Cushing's, called ectopic, and is crazy rare (surprise). Friends, the percentages they have shared bring no comfort to me given my last three medical years have all been in a world under five percent.

I have been medically intrigued as I watch this new doctor work with Dr. Kharlip and her team. It reminds me how lucky I am to have Dr. Kharlip as my captain because a lot of doctors just don't realize everything there is to know about Cushing's and how it can present itself. The back and forth among the specialists at the University of Pennsylvania is fascinating – it is also not lost on me that I understand more than sixty percent of their conversations. If an expert radiologist doesn't think it is growing like a Cushionoid tumor, Dr. Kharlip and I would feel more comfortable if we could biopsy. Simultaneously my ACTH cell count has continued to slightly increase over the past year (not alarmingly, but still increasing).

Since we were told that it cannot be biopsied, we scheduled the surgery for January 27. Then Christmas Eve, maybe they can biopsy it to the day after Christmas - still not sure they can do a thin needle biopsy. The same reasons exist on December 29, 2014 as they did in June 2013 about a biopsy:

a. They don't think they could get it because of the loca-
    tion - again the whole breathing thing getting in the way;

b. If they could, they are not certain they would be able to
    get a good sample because of the location so close to the
    lung wall and diaphragm; and

c. It could perforate my diaphragm and possibly collapse
    my lung.

Now, I know I won't hear anything until next week. If I have
confused you then you are probably right where I am and I have
been present for every conversation.

The main concern about the procedure is that it is major surgery
for someone with adrenals - throw my situation into it and it is
crappy. It will be very painful with many potential complications
and I will be out of it for a while - a very small portion of my lung
will be removed. The major risk, as it would be for any patient
with this surgery, is getting pneumonia. They explained that it
is painful to cough and clear the lungs.

We have not really shared this with anyone. We wanted to share
it with you – we know you will respect that (especially not Carter
and most of our family). I didn't want to bother anyone and felt
stupid that "here I am again with some crazy thing." I thought
I could just keep this in and I am sorry for being selfish and
bothering you all with it. I wanted you to know that I am OK
and I am not trying to be rude by not returning calls. As always,
Chris and my immediate family have been amazing. I hate what
it does to them.

Candidly, I am more at peace knowing that the tumor will more
than likely come out. I recognize that my new life is a little unusual but I get it and we live with it. We never know when the

other shoe will drop but I know my body well enough that I get a pretty good heads up. There are mostly great days with a few hurdles scattered in. I love working and continue to make an impact with clients I work with, but more importantly, try to be the best mom/wife/friend/daughter I can be. When the shoe does drop - I watch *Sex in the City* marathons, sleep, think of news ideas for next year's Cushing's fundraiser and figure out how to get on *Ellen*, on the *Today Show*, or in *People* magazine to bring awareness to this disease. Thank you for listening (reading). Please don't feel like you need to respond - I know you are praying for me and I will let you know what is going on when we know.

As I conclude this e-mail, please know that the lump that has been in my stomach is gone (I just wish the one in my lung was...)

From: Marie Conley
Sent: Monday, January 5, 2015 9:33 AM
Subject: Next Steps

Dr. Kharlip,

I hope the rest of your holiday was wonderful and that you were able to enjoy time off with your family. I cannot thank you enough for all that you have been doing for me these past couple of weeks. I recognize (which is a good thing) I am moving down on the priority level among your patients, which is a great feeling. I also don't mean to be overbearing or impatient about this next phase and continue to run to your side. I respect how valuable your time is, so I will try to articulate my thoughts in this e-mail. I have been doing some thinking and researching. I think I fully appreciate how complicated and painful this surgery would be. I also have faith that everything I have been told for the past nineteen months still holds true regarding the thin needle biopsy - it is not really possible; there are several risks that will more than likely not produce enough cells for a true sample. I have been told by Dr. Sun-Wo, her radiology team, Dr. Pechet and his team, that this wouldn't be possible. If it were, the last nineteen months of anguish would have been all for naught.

I think you know I always try to push through any bumps that may come in my path, but in my bones and gut I feel like I need to get this "thingie" out. I won't pretend to understand all of the medical terms or the percentages attached to it, but I know I don't find any resolve in the numbers. In nearly three years, I was assured I was not sick and told not to worry about it and the percentages of it being "anything" were slim to none. In the past two years since my diagnosis, I have lived in percentages that have been slim to none. For goodness sake, we tried for years to get pregnant and I am one of the few freaks that have permanent DI with a period.

While I have made most of my medical decisions based on facts involving little if any emotion, I need to acknowledge this is the first one where I am allowing "a feeling" to carry some weight. I can accept, not always understand, what has happened to me and remain thankful that I have the fortitude, family support, and faith to just keep moving forward. This situation with my lung is different. It never made sense; why was I the car accident a few weeks after by hernia operation? If it wasn't for that, I truly don't think this would have ever really come to light - at least at this time. Ironically, almost every other bone, organ, and blood count will be accounted for, for the rest of my life, but not my lungs.

I have accepted the unpredictable predictability of this disease, no adrenals, and the DI. I want a level playing field when it comes to my lungs. The spot was not there. It is there now and it is growing. The radiologists state it doesn't seem to be taking on particular characteristics, or it is slow growing. This doesn't provide a comfort I think I would have had if this were six years ago. Low percentages and normal characteristics have not been on my side before.

I believe this is where the ACTH cells are and I don't like the idea that maybe in a few years or as little as six months, we may be exactly where we are now. If the cells are there, I want them out of my body. You said I am strong enough to take this surgery on. I know you will work with Dr. Pechet and his team to make sure my endocrine side is managed well. I will write in permanent marker all over my body "I have no adrenals and DI" and to "please pay special attention to my fluids before, during, and after the surgery." I promise to walk around the minute I am allowed to and will do everything I am told.

Right now, I know you and your team are there. I know you trust Dr. Pechet. I trust the University of Pennsylvania hospital and I am strong. I am not comfortable looking for someone who will "agree" to do a procedure (the needle biopsy) when so many others already said no, then hope that they can actually do it and get a sample without puncturing a lung or diaphragm. You know my luck -- it will take me forever to heal from the biopsy and I will still need the surgery.

Please know I am not giving up. On the contrary, I believe I am taking a strategic approach to my health while doing what is best in the long run for my son and husband.

I would like to move forward with your blessing for Dr. Pechet to surgically remove the growth on January 27 and biopsy it.

Author's note: Sent to a larger group

From: Marie Conley
Sent: Friday, January 23, 2015 12:05 AM
Subject: Out damned spot.

Well friends, it has been a while since I have written about some new exciting path that my Cushing's journey has taken me on, but you know I am a giver and I feel you needed to have something new to shake your head about....

Some of you may remember in May 2013 I was in a fender bender (my fender was the one bent). While I hated being in the ambulance (precautionary only), there was no real damage from the accident. But it was during this trip to the ER that an X-ray showed an unusual spot on my lower right lobe lung. I went to Penn to see Dr. Kharlip and a great group of thoracic doctors who have been observing this little bugger for twenty months. On Dec. 19, I went back down for one of my routine visits and *yada yada yada*, the doctors (including my Captain) have decided it is time for it to come out.

NOW this wouldn't be me without a couple of little twists and turns.... You're probably thinking ---

> *"Marie, just get it biopsied."* Well, the doctors cannot biopsy. It is in such an "unusual" place near my diaphragm and lower right lung that it is not easily accessible. Or you're thinking – *"Just leave it in and deal with it later"* --- and in a way, we have. They have been monitoring it for twenty months now.

Quickly, the ACTH cells (or Cushing's causing cells) were never actually found when the biopsies came back from both the pituitary and adrenal surgeries (not unheard of for Cushing's because the sneaky buggers could be in the pituitary stalk or sinus cavity). Jump ahead to today --- this spot on my lung could be where these bugger cells are (this is called ectopic Cushing's). While it is unlikely, it could make sense, so we just need to be sure. The good news is the doctors really are not overly concerned about it either way.

SO.... on **Tuesday, January 27** early in the am, I will be in surgery getting this removed. It should take between two to four hours and they plan to do a video-assisted thorascopic surgery aka VATS. (For those counting, that will be a total of twelve holes in my abdomen thanks to Cushing's!) The location of the bugger makes the surgery a little tricky. My conditions (adrenal insufficient and the DI) and the fact that a small piece of my lung will be extracted from my body, make this procedure pretty crappy. (Then again, what's a little sliver of lung, when HUP already has my adrenals and a piece of my pituitary?)

I will be at Penn Presbyterian Center (finally, a change of location). I am under the care of one of the best surgeons, Dr. Taine Pechet and my captain, Dr. Julia Kharlip. I have FULL faith in their hands and in God's path for me. Chris is a complete pillar of strength and laughter (apparently I will heal better if we have a larger smart TV in our bedroom); Carter is nothing short of amazing – he is smarter and wiser than most adults are. His questions and concerns are thoughtful and sensitive, but like his father, he adds a bit of humor to it as well. My mom, dad, sister, as well as the small group we shared this with have been so supportive throughout these past few weeks. We have been going back and forth with the doctors throughout the holiday SO I am very sorry that so many of you are finding out through e-mail. This should explain why I have been off the grid for the past month.

They say I should only be in the hospital for four to five days (you should have heard me giggle at that one.) Chris and Carter will be in Philly with me for Tuesday and Wednesday. Then it is home for three weeks of recovery. Given the location of the bugger, my medical history, and the possible complications (and the doctors' orders) will truly leave me homebound. Nurse Babci (aka my mom) will be with us and I promise that we will lean on you for help when we need it.

I have matured medically, personally, spiritually, and professionally since this started in 2012. I know we cannot do this alone. It is OK to share that I have a crappy disease. Because of Sue and Scott Paterno and a few other clients, I continue to work and help make an impact. I hope to be back to answering e-mails and being on calls within two weeks. I recognize and never question that God has put me on this path for a reason and that good will come out of it. Case in point, with all of your help, in November we raised over $35,000 that will go toward supporting research, awareness, and healing about this disease. In fact, I already met with the development folks and Dr. Kharlip, important research will be started with these funds (and it was a great excuse to hold a party --- look for your 'Kickin' Cushing's to the Curb' ~ *Fiesta Style* invite on November 13, 2015). Hershey Entertainment & Resorts has agreed to be a key sponsor!

I will continue to kick this thing's butt. I have already signed up for a 10K and a Sprint Triathlon for late spring/early summer – and while I may not finish them – I will try my hardest to be at the starting line! I know you are praying for me but please send a few extra more Carter's way. Apparently, I will be on some pretty strong meds so I will e-mail and call when I can. While I did get a subscription to Amazon Prime and Netflix, I would eventually love some company for those who are local.

Chris will send an e-mail out next Tuesday to let you know that it went well. Thank you all for everything you have done to get us this far...

Sent to the Board, Presidents and staff of the Pennsylvania State System of Higher Education. I have been a member of the Board of Governor's since 2003.

From: Marie Conley
Sent: Friday, January 23, 2015 12:50 AM
Subject: Upcoming weeks

It was great to see many of you today. I wanted to let you know that I will be "off the grid" for the next couple of weeks.

On Tuesday, I will be having surgery (again) – this time on my right lower lung area. For the past 20 months, the docs at Penn have been monitoring a spot on my lung. Over the holiday, it was decided that it is time to take it out and see what is going on. Though we think this is probably Cushing's-related and no one is overly concerned (or sure!), the surgery is just a bit rough and we need to be extra careful due to my medical baggage (clearly not a medical term).

I will be at Penn Presbyterian for about five days, then back to Hershey to recover. I have spoken to Guido and Kathleen about my participation over the next three to four weeks. I was told to prepare for a tough recovery and while I have no doubt I will be back in fighting shape soon, I am probably going to (try) to listen to the doctors this time (ha ha).

I will answer e-mails when I am able and participate via conference calls. I am definitely homebound for three weeks after I return from the hospital. I know I am in great hands and have the best medical team surrounding me. God is also having too much fun with me so I know I am OK in His book. Most importantly, Carter is handling this with a level of maturity and humor well past his almost 10 years.

Chris will reach out to Audrey to keep you in the loop after the surgery. Please keep us in your thoughts.

From: Marie Conley
Sent: Tuesday, January 27, 2015 3:57 PM
Subject: Marie Update

Friends,

As the saying goes, "the third time's the charm." I am happy to report that the third (and hopefully final!!) Cushing's-related surgery went well today. Not only was the surgeon able to remove the growth on Marie's lung, but all is going well in recovery. Marie's team of very caring doctors was able to keep her blood and sodium levels from fluctuating wildly, which had been the source of so many post-surgery challenges in the past.

As you can imagine, Marie is in a normal amount of pain for the procedure. However, I think we are beginning to realize how even the slightest shifts in the body result in the movement of the lungs. Needless to say, she is limiting her movements because even under serious pain medications, it is not a pleasant feeling.

Thank you for your kind words of support throughout this entire journey.

Chris (for Marie)

From: Marie Conley
Sent: Thursday, February 5, 2015 10:34 PM
Subject: So I lied.... sort of

A funny thing happened on my journey to Kickin' Cushing's to the Curb – I got a hard detour back in the hospital on Tuesday morning; hence, I am sorry to those I have not thanked or reached out to since my e-mail on Saturday.

On Monday, I started to feel a little weird. (yes, I will pause so you may insert your own joke) Anyway, at 8:00 am Tuesday, I was getting bloodwork run for Dr. Kharlip and by noon I was in the ER and admitted; blessed with another beautifully woven little moon and stars hospital gown; had ten-plus blood draws, and 32 hours later was released! While at Penn State Hershey Medical Center, I was under the care of Dr. Kharlip at University of Pennsylvania and a good team at PSHMC and discharged last night at 7:30 pm. It was probably a combination of pain from the lung procedure -meets –adrenal- crisis -meets sodium crash or vice versa, but due to the lack of cooperation between my many disorders, I landed back in the hospital. Thank goodness, my mom was here. Dr. Kharlip is tweaking my medications and is monitoring my 'I' and 'O's for the next week. (Ins and outs of what I am drinking and peeing; that's for you and me, Russ)

I hope you don't mind my sharing, but I promised to keep you up to date. I also thought you would appreciate this morning's task: I created a one-page Excel spreadsheet that lists all of my medications, dosages, and time schedules, because if I had to articulate ONE MORE TIME my medications, dosages, and time schedules to one more doctor, nurse, resident, or medical student I was going to freak out. I now have a one page color coded chart to distribute in case this happens again in the next two weeks. (I also included footnotes for those reviewing it who are not familiar with the diseases or subsequent surgeries and side effects)

Yes, my friends, I am back (at least getting there) but I promise I will continue to listen to doctors' (*and* my Mommy's *and* Chris's *and* Carter's) orders and rest.

From: Marie Conley
Sent: Monday, February 23, 2015 12:32 AM
Subject: Marie Update -

I hope this e-mail finds you all well.

Chris, Carter, and I wanted to thank you so very much for all you have done for us these past three and a half weeks. Many reached out over the weekend to find out how my follow-up doctor's appointment went last week with my thoracic surgeon. I haven't gotten back to you yet because I needed to change the appointment. I decided I would like to hang out at Penn State Hershey Medical Center again, so I had Chris bring me to the ER on Thursday morning and I have been in here ever since. For those counting, this is my second time here since the chest surgery (down at Penn January 27 – back home January 31- admitted to Penn State Hershey on Tuesday, February 3 – back home the night of the 4 and back to the Med Center Feb. 19 where I am now).

There is just something about me and these awesome hospital gowns!

We think it was another adrenal crisis. (If I have this correct) I think I can explain what is happening by saying the internal healing in my body for the chest surgery is causing "stress" that is using my hydrocortisone meds (steroids). I probably wasn't compensating enough with oral pain medication because I wasn't feeling the physical pain/stress, so my body was fighting over the hydrocortisone to relieve that "stress" and cover what it needed for my normal every day activities. There is a secret formula to keeping the right level of hydrocortisone, my sodium, and electrolytes needed to stay balanced in my body on a normal day in addition to aiding it along when there are added stresses – whether I feel them or not. Because I do not have adrenal glands and I have the permanent DI (diabetes insipidus) – it makes it a little extra tricky. The doctors are working on that secret formula. The irony is not lost on me that I need to articulate and differentiate between different levels of stress–Hello, TYPE A.

I thought I was busting out today but my numbers dipped again so I remain here. I want to believe I am getting out tomorrow but I know better than to believe it is true until I feel the discharge papers in my hand. As always, Captain Kharlip at University of Pennsylvania is part of the crew steering the ship. The plus side is I had a beautiful view of the snow yesterday outside of my window. My "office" has been set up since Friday, and I am working here as if I were at home. I have the kindest nursing team and endocrine doctors at Penn State Hershey and am lucky enough to have snuggle time at night with Carter, and romantic florescent- lighted strolls in antiseptic-filled hallways of Penn State Hershey Medical sixth floor with Chris. However, I will be honest and admit I am now over this; I want to be done with this detour. I have been stressed- dosed with steroids for more than twenty-eight days – my face is crazy puffy, my body is a mess, as I have, yet again, gained weight without the joy of earning those calories through cream-filled donuts, fries, or real sour cream on nachos. I haven't driven or really even been out in public since January 26. I am so sick of *Law and Order* and *NCIS* marathons.

As always, (and not unexpectedly), I have taken an active participatory role in my care as I am the only constant and the endocrine world is a mystery. While I would prefer not to be here, and am resentful of the time that has been taken away from my life with my family, I know how lucky I am. I remember meeting a miracle child at Children's Miracle Network, Eli Sidler. His was one of my first families. He was diagnosed with a rare bone cancer and died in 2012. His memorial was the day before my first brain surgery. I remember his father saying, "Eli had cancer, cancer didn't have Eli." I have tried to live my life remembering those words every day through the ups and downs.

I have Cushing's –Cushing's does NOT have ME. I will not let it win. My parents raised me better than that, and Chris and I want to raise Carter to be better than letting something like this define him. I have made an active choice to be defined by the type of mother, daughter, wife, sister, friend and colleague that I am.

I believe that the work I do is effective and makes an impact. I want to be defined by what I have chosen to do: to use my God-given talents and skills, and take the negativity of this disease, turn it around, and create something positive. I want to create awareness and healing for those burdened with Cushing's. I want to help their families and friends understand the disease for what it is. I want to help them survive.

While I go back to Penn March 4 to have my follow-up from the surgery, I have been told that they found neither ACTH nor malignant producing cells in the little bugger in my lung. That is great news and I will be given the full breakdown when I see my surgeon. If it is anything other than boring medical stuff, I will keep you posted, but knowing what it is or isn't puts me back on my version of a level playing field. We wouldn't have known this if we didn't have this surgery.

We have many things to look forward to over the next couple of months. Carter heads to Universal Studios with my sister on Thursday and will be meeting my parents there for four days. I hope to work on some awareness opportunities with the University of Pennsylvania Hospital in April for National Cushing's Awareness Day (April 8) and Chris is over the moon that the legislature is in for the next two weeks! I have twenty-eight weeks until the Hershey Half. It is about having a tangible goal and trying to achieve it. I may not run across the finish line gracefully (or maybe not at all), but I will definitely be at the start!

We can't wait to see you all and feel so lucky to have such great friends and family.

From: Marie Conley
Sent: Monday, February 23, 2015 10:08 PM
Subject: I'm home.

That's all. Just sooo happy.

We are so lucky to have you in our lives – your good wishes and prayers got me home tonight.

Good-bye for now.

From: Marie Conley
Sent: Monday, June 1, 2015 7:14 PM
Subject: Cushing's Update

Howdy. I know it has been a while since my last e-mail. I have started this e-mail so many times in the past month; I just haven't been able to actually finish it. I usually have some funny experience or some freaky story to share with you on this journey, but I have been stumped lately. I think that is why I have been hesitant to write.

For the most part, it hasn't been all that bad since the lung surgery in January but I can't say that it wasn't a bit bumpy since the end of February. I have been back and forth to doctor appointments here & in Philly. I have had about six different infections which led me to about four different antibiotics, medication changes (additions and subtractions), blood pressure monitoring, blood draws, weight gain (thank you steroids), night sweats, something wrong with the ligaments in my jaw, thinning hair and oh, yeah, tested positive Epstein-Barr (this is like mono) and was back in PT through early May. In mid-March and April, I was experiencing the cognitive challenges at times that I have always read about. It scared the living crap outta' me. My body was basically rebooting and there was nothing I could do. Dr. Kharlip assured me it would get better; I just had to be patient. Chris and I have just had to laugh sometimes through my tears. For the first time since I was diagnosed in 2012, I felt like maybe this was getting the better of me. When I tell you I couldn't wait for spring, I was not kidding.

In March, our Cushing's Support Group that I started met again. Our numbers have grown, there are now seven of us able to attend gatherings and another five that are involved through e-mail. Most of us are University of Penn patients in the tristate area. I have come to cherish this time with them and feel a level of peace for those two hours that I don't usually have. I think it is because no one has to say a word, but we all understand each other. It also has reminded me how truly blessed I am because I am one of the really healthy ones and more importantly, I am surrounded by such a strong circle of family and friends. To see what some of the others are going through really shook me. It also reinforced how lucky I am to have you and how important it is to make sure those of us who aren't alone can reach out to others in need who have Cushing's.

I think that is why the past three months have been difficult for me to adjust to as well as reach out to you. Realities of the level of vulnerabilities I experienced that are common for individuals who have (had) Cushing's really got to me. For the past three months, I have focused on being everything I could be for Carter and my home; being successful at work, and then crashing. I have had bursts of energy - some of you have been on the receiving end of what I refer to as "drive by" calls. I phone - then when you call back, I enter radio silence mode – not on purpose, but by then I've become exhausted. I haven't been a very good friend lately and I am sorry for that. Dr. Kharlip has cleared me for the next three months – we are working on a new medication regimen and it has only been the last two to three weeks that I am starting to feel like myself again.

Laying low is a self-inflicting isolation that I cannot let myself continue to experience. I wanted to wait to reach out until I felt like my old self. I cannot hide as I have until I "feel better or feel like myself" because Chris and I have come to realize that "feeling better" is all relative. I am even more resolved to make sure that whatever I do – be it work or play – is meaningful and memorable. What makes me feel better - "like myself" - is laughing and being around the people I care about, so be prepared for some friendship and family stalking... I have to make up for lost time!

So there it is. I will keep on keeping on. I continue to work with Dr. Kharlip and the Development team at Penn. Funding from The Conley's Cushing's Fund will soon be granted to an important research project at the University of Pennsylvania for Cushing's patients. Some money has been invested on working on a few publications for families and friends who have Cushing's patients in their lives and a children's book. We are continuing to grow the Cushing's support group. We are planning for the BEST birthday bash ever.... Friday, November 13 Kickin' Cushing's to the Curb ~ *Fiesta style*. It is so important to keep the awareness of this disease out there.

I am trying to be the best person I can be: remembering that I have Cushing's disease, but Cushing's does not have me; and to embrace the present!

PS: It is not a Cushing's e-mail without one bizarre story --- as you know, the biopsy from my lung was NOT the Cushing's thingie ---- it ended up being some rare spore that is predominantly found in the Mississippi Delta (or something like that) or if you check WebMD – sometimes in bat caves. For the record, I have never been to the Mississippi Delta (wherever that is...) and I have never been in a cave. REALLY ---- Bats!

AFTERWORD

Cushing's disease and the complications that come from it are a part of my daily life. A week after the last e-mail, I was rushed to the ER for an adrenal crisis. In July, I started to see a reproductive endocrinologist to help navigate hormonal imbalances that have started to occur. I need to take a few additional medications (none of which have a side effect of weight loss.) That is just how the cookie is going to crumble. I have good days and bad days. Who doesn't?

What really matters is my family had a great time in Bethany Beach in August and I watched my son's face as he saw his first Boston Red Sox game at Fenway Park. On good days, I am running five to seven miles in my quest to cross the finish line at the Hershey Half Marathon on October 18. I may be pacing a 13:30 mile and this will probably be my last long distance race but Cushing's will not deny me this goal.

Our support group continues to meet and we have grown by a few. Those few hours together every couple months means so much to me.

Lastly, we are in the final stages for planning the second annual Kickin' Cushing's to the Curb *Fiesta Style* in November. All dollars raised will continue to support The Conley Cushing's Disease Fund. We will have great food, margaritas flowing from multiple directions, a demonstration of hand rolled cigars will be available for the guests and music that will make everyone dance.

If you are going to have a crappy disease, you might as well have a good party!

ABOUT THE AUTHOR

Marie Conley is a consultant focusing on engagement and stakeholder strategies and fund development for a variety of clients through her company Conley Consulting, LLC.

During her tenure in politics (1994-2009), Marie was a trusted advisor to top-level government officials and private sector organizations beginning in 1994 as the scheduler to Governor Tom Ridge. In 2009, as a senior level fundraiser, strategist and event planner, she made a successful transition from Pennsylvania's highly competitive political landscape into the equally challenging field of non-profit development as director of Penn State Hershey's Children's Miracle Network. Since 2012, her focus has been working with Sue Paterno, wife the late Coach Joe Paterno, to assist with a number of initiatives around the issue of prevention and awareness of child sexual victimization.

Marie never takes any professional or personal task at face value. She is always looking for ways to improve efficiencies, outcomes and most importantly calls upon herself and those around her to do the right thing for the right reasons. Her accomplishments in such a short period of time at Children's Miracle Network are only one example.

Marie serves as the Vice Chairman for the Board of Governor member of the Pennsylvania State System of Higher Education.

She is Chair of the Academic and Student Affairs Committee and has spearheaded significant changes in policy regarding the recruitment and hiring practices for university presidential and chancellor searches and has re-evaluated and changed the policy for university presidential evaluations. Marie was first nominated in 2002 by Governor Mark Schweiker; was re-appointed by Governor Ed Rendell in 2004 and re-appointed by Governor Tom Corbett in 2012. From 1997 to 2011, Marie served as a Council of Trustee for her alma mater, Bloomsburg University of Pennsylvania. Marie volunteers at St. Joan of Arc School.

In 2012, Marie was diagnosed with a rare disease called Cushing's disease. Cushing's disease is so unusual that it affects less than ten people per million each year. On July 17, 2014, The Conley Cushing's Disease Fund was established and is a project of The Foundation for Enhancing Communities, fiscal sponsor. The funds raised will be used in part to create awareness materials for loved ones who are suffering from this disease as well support institutions and organizations focused on issues surrounding Cushing's disease. She has committed her talents and gifts to raise money and awareness for those with Cushing's disease and complications from the disease.

Marie hails from Bucks County, Pennsylvania; she lives outside Hershey, Pennsylvania with her husband, Chris Lammando, and their ten year old son, Carter.

www.ingramcontent.com/pod-product-compliance
Lightning Source LLC
Chambersburg PA
CBHW030350290526
45785CB00004B/1675